HEALTHY HEART
SOUTH ASIAN DIET

Healthy Heart South Asian Diet

Lalita Kaul
PhD, RD, LDN.
Professor of Nutrition
Department of Community Health and Family Practice
College of Medicine
Howard University, Washington, D.C.

SEABOARD PRESS
AN IMPRINT OF J. A. ROCK & CO., PUBLISHERS

Healthy Heart South Asian Diet by Lalita Kaul

SEABOARD PRESS

is an imprint of *JAMES A. ROCK & CO., PUBLISHERS*

Address comments and inquiries to:
SEABOARD PRESS
9710 Traville Gateway Drive, #305
Rockville, MD 20850

E-mail:
jrock@rockpublishing.com lrock@rockpublishing.com
Internet URL: www.rockpublishing.com

Paperback ISBN: 1-59663-756-0

Library of Congress Control Number: 2006920027

Printed in the United States of America

First Edition: 2006

Dedicated

to

Janki Nath Ganju

ACKNOWLEDGMENTS

My special thanks go to Ms. Ruth Matthews for her assistance in putting the book manuscript together. I am grateful for the support of my husband, Dr. Dali J. Patel, and my daughter, Kavita Patel, who stimulated me enormously in this project. And finally, I am grateful for the support and love of my mother, Mrs. Aruna Kaul, and my brother, Maharaj Krishen Kaul.

Lalita Kaul

Table of Contents

Tables

FOREWORD

More than a million people living in the United States trace their origin to South Asia. Many are doctors, engineers, scientists, and teachers — in short, members of highly demanding professions whose requirements for membership are intelligence, education and motivation. Yet, ironically, this immigrant generation finds itself increasingly prone to developing heart disease at a time when the general American population is making substantial progress in halting and even reducing this life-threatening condition. Perhaps the increase in heart disease among Asian Americans is due to the ease with which our adopted country allows us to fulfill our craving for traditionally rich, fatty South Asian foods as well as other deleterious ingestibles such as smoking and alcohol. Moreover, recent health-related research shows that blood lipid abnormalities present in South Asian communities are substantially different from those in the typical American community. The major lipid abnormality among Americans in general is: elevated levels of low density lipoprotein (LDL) cholesterol, in contrast to the Asian Americans where the major abnormality is elevated triglyceride levels, low high density lipoprotein (HDL) levels and only minimally elevated LDL cholesterol level.

The risk factors for heart disease are well-established. The main contributors are rich and fatty diets, lack of exercise and smoking. Genetic factors also play a significant role. Add to this a tendency toward a sedentary lifestyle, obesity, diabetes, hypertension and occupational stresses in the population, and one can see a prescription for a major heart attack. To significantly decrease their chances of developing heart disease, they need to adapt a healthier lifestyle that includes an appropriate diet, exercise, abstinence from smoking and adequate weight control. The choice is theirs if they want to increase the length and fullness of their life.

This book is written to inform and motivate Asian Americans toward the choice of a healthy heart diet. The author, Dr. Lalita Kaul, is an authority and activist in communicating the need for lifestyle changes among Asians. She has treated a large number of Asian patients, but through this book and her lectures to medical students at Howard University College of Medicine in Washington, DC, she seeks to reach more people.

Her goal is to accomplish three major objectives:

(1) Provide a definition of the various risk factors for heart disease as they pertain to Americans of South Asian origin.
(2) Establish the importance of a healthy heart diet for this community and all others who are ***"hooked"*** on rich South Asian foods.
(3) Develop and illustrate a heart diet based on "appropriate" foods, i.e., substitute dishes that will still be enjoyable to persons who now maintain a typical South Asian diet.

If the food substitutions discussed in this book are adopted, they will lower cholesterol levels, reduce triglyceride levels and increase HDL levels — all indicators of a healthy heart. They can accomplish this without sacrificing the well-loved tastes of their favorite Asian dishes.

It must be emphasized that diet alone is not a magic protection against heart disease. Regular exercise, total abstinence from smoking (including secondary inhalation from those who remain addicted to nicotine), moderation in alcohol intake, a reduction of occupational stress factors and proper control of diabetes and/or hypertension are also necessary. All of these disciplines must be maintained in a discipline tandem if results are to be achieved.

But first in importance is a healthy heart diet — an essential beginning in achieving a changed lifestyle. Physically and psychologically, it is the first giant step toward a renewed and fulfilling longer life.

Dali J. Patel, MD, PhD

PREFACE

Let's face it. Eating is one of the great pleasures of life.

However, too much of the wrong foods can lead to obesity, diabetes, high blood pressure, heart disease and stroke. The 2003 United States Surgeon General's Report on Health and Nutrition underscores the importance of diet in achieving and maintaining a healthy life. It concludes that ***"over consumption of certain dietary components is now a major concern for Americans. While many food factors are involved, chief among them is the disproportionate consumption of foods high in fats, often at the expense of foods high in complex carbohydrates and fiber that may be more conducive to health."*** Fortunately, we all have the power to achieve and maintain good health by making the right choices in the foods that we eat. The Surgeon General's report recommends that a healthy diet should contain foods that will ensure proper weight and circulatory maintenance through the significant reduction of fat — especially saturated fat — as well as reductions of cholesterol, sugar and sodium. The report also emphasizes the need to increase fiber to obtain improved dietary results. And it states that alcohol intake should always be moderate. Although many Americans have changed their diets from the unhealthy pattern that existed during studies made in the 1970s, too many Asian Americans of the past two decades have retained bad eating habits. They have exchanged their originally **moderate average** dietary intake of total fat, saturated fat, polyunsaturated fat and cholesterol for a diet that **virtually assures** a rise in their overall rate of heart disease.

In addition to over-consumption of saturated fats and simple sugars, it is suggested that some Asians may have a gene which makes them more prone to develop coronary artery disease. The discovery that gene predisposes certain individuals to heart disease was made by researchers at the University of California at Berkeley. The gene is classic because by itself it does not cause atherosclerosis, but when teamed with other factors, like diet, and other genes, it puts an individual at greater risk of developing heart disease. For many Asians, an interaction of this ***"heart disease"*** gene with environmental factor, like diet can be a life threatening scenario. This may account for the increase of premature coronary artery disease among South Asians in the United States.

This book recognizes the special needs of people raised in the traditional cultures of South Asia, but offers a way of achieving a more balanced diet that will greatly reduce a tendency to becoming overweight and at the same time will reduce coronary artery disease. The book also tries to achieve these goals in the least painful way to achieve maximum compliance. After all, one is dealing with life long dietary habits which need to be altered permanently.

After explaining the risk factors in heart disease (Chapters 1,2 3) and the peculiarities of heart disease patterns in South Asians (Chapter 4), one turns to more practical aspects of the problem. Chapter 5 and 6 will help the person select proper foods from grocery stores, etc. Chapter 7 on "eating out" has many practical hints that will minimize "damage" for a population that enjoys eating out especially those households in which both husband and wife work. Chapter 8, together with the recipe-modification section and the tables, will provide many ingenious ideas for substitutions that will make eating at home a pleasure with no associated guilt. These recipes are designed to reduce the amount of saturated fat, salt and total calories from the original dish, with essentially no alteration in TASTE, that could even fool the experts. This demonstrates the general philosophy of the author that, *"even half a loaf is better than no loaf at all"*.

Lalita Kaul, PhD, RD, LDN

CHAPTER 1

RISK FACTORS FOR CARDIOVASCULAR DISEASE

Risk factors are associated with an increased likelihood of developing a disease. Risk factors may be laboratory measurements, such as serum low-density lipoprotein (LDL) cholesterol or high-density lipoprotein (HDL) cholesterol, or physical exam measurements, such as blood pressure, or habits such as cigarette smoking. Risk factors for cardiovascular disease (CVD) are classified as either controllable, which means they are amenable to modification or noncontrollable. For example, high blood pressure and LDL cholesterol can be treated with medication, whereas age and family history cannot be changed. Cardiovascular disease is identified by the third Adult Treatment Panel of the National Cholesterol Education Program (ATP III).

When examining risk factors for coronary heart disease (CHD), it is important to understand the atherosclerotic process because each risk factor contributes to plaque formation. Theories for the pathophysiology of atherosclerosis include vascular injury, and viral or bacterial infection, but the most widely accepted is the lipid infiltration hypothesis. Excess LDL can become oxidized and taken up in various tissues by scavenger receptors.

Controllable and Non-Controllable Cardiovascular Disease Risk Factors

Controllable Factors	Non-controllable Factors
Cigarette smoking Hypertension (blood pressure >120/80 mm Hg Dyslipidemia Diabetes mellitus Obesity Physical inactivity	increasing age (men > 45 years: women >55 years) Family history of premature CHD (male first=degree relative <55 years, female first-degree relative <65years)

Many enzymes that function in normal cell processes produce free radicals that can oxidize LDL. Such enzymes include NADPH oxidase, 15-lipoxygenase, myeloperoxidase, and the mitochrondrial electron transport system. All of these enzymes are active during normal cell metabolism. During an inflammatory response, as occurs in the atherosclerotic lesion, even more free radicals are produced. Environmental factors, such as cigarette smoking, increase the amount of free radicals in the circulation and increase the risk of oxidation. Genetic conditions, such as high homocysteine levels due to inefficient methionine metabolism, can also cause oxidative damage to LDL.

LDL CHOLESTEROL

Risk factors for atherosclerosis include smoking, high blood pressure, and diabetes, all of which can damage the arterial wall and increase production of free radicals. In addition, genetic factors such as defects in the LDL receptor, presence of apoliproprotein B or E, and presence of lipoprotein lipase increase the risk for atherosclerosis because these deficiencies cause a great increase in plasma LDL cholesterol. A diet high in saturated fat and a sedentary lifestyle also increase plasma LDL cholesterol and the risk for atherosclerosis.

The risk for coronary artery disease can be reduced with a low-fat diet and regular exercise, both of which are known to reduce plasma LDL cholesterol levels. In addition, regular consumption of food containing vitamins with antioxidant properties can reduce the amount of free radicals available to oxidize LDL. Adding fiber to the diet can increase loss of cholesterol through the intestine and help maintain cholesterol homeostasis in the body. Finally, high levels of HDL cholesterol are inversely correlated with the risk for heart disease. HDL has been shown to be protective in several ways. It may have antioxidant properties and, thus, prevent oxidation of LDL. In addition, it has been shown to reduce the growth and migration of smooth muscle cells and inhibit adhesion of monocytes to endothelial cells. HDL is the major lipoprotein involved in the process of reverse cholesterol transport where cholesterol is removed from peripheral cells and returned to the liver for catabolism, thus preventing an overaccumulation of cholesterol in the tissues.

Evidence for LDL cholesterol as the main contributor to CHD have been shown by epidemiologic, animal, cell, and biochemical studies, as well as human population studies and clinical trials. An example is the genetic mutation of the LDL receptor that causes familial hypercholesterolemia, a condition that causes accelerated atherosclerosis in humans. In addition, animal models in which the LDL receptor is defective show the development of atherosclerosis in animals that do not normally develop coronary lesions.

Population studies, such as the Framingham Heart Study, Multiple Risk Factor Intervention Trial (MRFIT), and the Lipid Research Clinics Study (LRC), have shown a direct relationship between LDL cholesterol level (or total cholesterol) and new onset CHD in both men and women initially free of CHD. In the MRFIT trial of 12,866 high-risk men, subjects randomized to clinical intervention had a 7.5% decrease in total cholesterol and a 15% decrease in CHD incidence compared with subjects randomized to usual care after a 6-year follow-up. Therefore, a 1% reduction in serum cholesterol level yielded a 2% reduction in the risk of CHD.

Populations with higher LDL cholesterol levels have more atherosclerosis than populations with lower LDL cholesterol levels. To determine whether diet or genetics is a more important predictor in populations, Japanese men living in three locations were compared in the Ni-Hon-San Study. Dietary saturated fat intake was 7% in Japanese men living in Japan, 12% in Japanese men living in Hawaii, and 14% in Japanese men living in San Francisco. Serum cholesterol correlated with saturated fat intake with the lowest levels in Japan and highest levels in San Francisco. Death rates from CHD were1.7 times higher in Hawaii and 2.8 times greater in San Francisco than in Japan. Therefore, diet appears to be a more important factor than genetics.

Recent studies have shown that high cholesterol levels in early youth can predict the development of CHD later in life. Long-term follow-up in three prospective studies showed that increased cholesterol levels in early adulthood were associated with increased risk for CHD in middle age. In contrast, populations with total cholesterol levels less than 150 mg/dL or LDL cholesterol levels less than 100 mg/dL throughout life have almost no clinical CHD. Therefore, starting intervention for high LDL cholesterol early in life is important for prevention.

A review of numerous statin trials (3-hydroxy-3-methylglutaryl coenzyme A [HMG-CoA] reductase inhibitors) showed that CHD mortality and total mortality were reduced with LDL cholesterol reduction. Several of these studies showed favorable changes in lesion architecture through coronary angiography with LDL cholesterol lowering. Statins were associated with reduction of CHD in both elderly and younger subjects, men and women, individuals with and without heart disease, individuals with and without diabetes, hypertensives and normotensives, and at most cholesterol levels.

Cigarette Smoking

Cigarette smoking is a potent contributor to risk for CHD and other forms of CVD. Smokers have double or triple the risk of myocardial infarction (MI) or fatal CHD as compared with nonsmokers. The risk increases with number of cigarettes smoked each day. For instance, heavy smokers have six times the risk of MI or fatal CHD as compared with nonsmokers. Smoking decreases HDL cholesterol levels and increases lipid oxidation, which, in turn, leads to uptake of excess cholesterol into the arteries by scavenger receptors. Data suggest cardiovascular benefits occur within months of quitting. Randomized clinical trials of smoking cessation have also shown substantial reduction in risk for cardiac events in those who quit. Within 2 years of quitting, women who smoked reduced their CHD risk to levels of women who never smoked.

Hypertension

A continuous relationship exists between blood pressure and risk of CVD – the higher the blood pressure, the higher the risk of MI, stroke, heart failure, and kidney disease. High blood pressure, or hypertension, is a risk factor for coronary heart disease. Obesity, lack of exercise, alcohol, smoking and stress are associated with hypertension in those with a predisposition to heart disease. Twenty-five to fifty percent of elevated blood pressure is due to genetics. The rest is caused by diet, lifestyle habits, physical activity and stress. The interaction between genes and environmental factors is not clear.

Classification Of Blood Pressure In Adults

RANGE, mm/Hg	CATEGORY
Diastolic	
< 80	Normal Blood Pressure
80 – 89	Prehypertension
90 – 99	Moderate hypertension
>100	Severe hypertension
Systolic, blood pressure	
under 120 – 89	Normal blood pressure
120 – 139	Prehypertension
140 –159	Borderline systolic hypertension
over 160	Systolic hypertension

The Framingham Heart Study has shown that subjects with blood pressure of 130/80 to 139/89 mm Hg are twice as likely to progress to hypertension than those with lower values. High normal blood pressure is associated with increased risk for CHD. On the basis of these studies, the latest Joint National Committee on Prevention, Detection, Evaluation, and Treatment of High Blood Pressure guidelines (JNC 7) introduced a new classification of prehypertension as systolic blood pressure of 120 to 139 mm Hg or diastolic blood pressure of 80 to 89 mm Hg. Subjects with prehypertension should be counseled on lifestyle modifications to prevent CVD.

Clinical trial evidence that blood pressure reduction decreases CHD endpoints provides further support of hypertension as a major risk factor. Antihypertensive therapy in clinical trials has been associated with a 20% to 25% reduction in MI, 35% to 40% reduction in stroke, and more than 50% reduction in heart failure.

Total Cholesterol

Cholesterol is a fat-like substance that is a main component of cell membranes. It is a precursor of bile acids and steroid hormones. The body automatically produces about 80-85 percent of total cholesterol, and the rest comes from the diet. The cholesterol level in blood plasma is determined partly by inheritance and partly by the fat and cholesterol content of the individual's diet. Americans consume about 300 to 600 milligrams daily. The National Cholesterol Education Program has set a maximum of 300 milligrams a day.

High blood cholesterol is one of the major factors in CHD. The risk of developing CHD increases as the blood cholesterol levels rise. Three categories of blood cholesterol levels have been defined by the National Institute of Health's Adult Treatment Panel as shown below:

Desirable	**High**	**Very High**
Blood Cholesterol	Blood Cholesterol	Blood Cholesterol
Less than 200 mg/dl	200-239 mg/dl	240 mg/dl and above

When a high blood cholesterol level is combined with another major risk factor (either high blood pressure or cigarette smoking), the risk for CHD increases even further. For example, if the cholesterol level is in the *"very high"* category and there is hypertension, the risk for CHD increases six times. Smoking increases the risk more than twenty times. Most CHD is caused by atherosclerosis, which occurs when cholesterol, fat, and other substances deposit in the walls of the arteries that supply blood to the heart. These deposits can slow or block the flow of blood and oxygen. Insufficient oxygen weakens the heart muscle, resulting in chest pain (angina), and a heart attack (myocardial infarction).

Lowering high blood cholesterol level will slow fatty build up in the arteries and reduce the risk of heart attack. Studies have shown that for each one percent reduction in total cholesterol levels, there is a 2 percent reduction in heart attacks. For example, if you reduce your cholesterol level by 10 percent, risk of coronary heart disease could drop by 20 percent. Some of the factors that influence blood cholesterol levels are as follows:

1. *Diet*: Saturated fat and dietary cholesterol raise blood cholesterol

2. *Weight*: Obesity may increase cholesterol level. Losing weight can help lower blood cholesterol level

3. *Exercise*: Regular exercise can increase HDL (good type of cholesterol)

4. *Genetic factors*: A small number of people have a genetic disorder that contributes to a high blood cholesterol level. These people require cholesterol lowering drugs.

HDL Cholesterol

Based on epidemiologic studies, low HDL cholesterol (< 40 mg/dL) is an independent risk factor for CHD after adjustment for other risk variables. High HDL cholesterol is associated with decreased risk for CHD. These studies have shown that a 1% decrease in HDL cholesterol yields a 2% to 3% increase in CHD risk. Some genetic forms of HDL deficiency increase the risk of CHD, whereas others do not. Genetic causes account for approximately 50% of variation in HDL cholesterol levels.

For certain populations, HDL cholesterol levels may be a better predictor for CVD than LDL cholesterol levels. For example, compared with an LDL cholesterol level less than 140 mg/dL, an LDL cholesterol level greater than 160 mg/dL is a weaker predictor of CHD risk in women age 65 years or older than in men. In contrast, compared with an HDL cholesterol greater than 60 mg/dL, an HDL cholesterol level less than 50 doubled the risk of death from CHD in women younger than 65 years. In addition, HDL cholesterol was the strongest predictor of CHD risk in four large epidemiologic studies. Furthermore, in men and women older than age 85, HDL cholesterol levels predict CHD mortality better than LDL cholesterol levels, which may be because subjects with high LDL cholesterol levels had already died from CHD.

Low levels of HDL cholesterol are associated with other atherogenic lipid factors, such as high triglyceride levels, remnant lipoproteins, and small dense LDL.

Several trials have shown that statins have more benefits in subjects with low levels of HDL cholesterol compared with subjects with higher levels of HDL cholesterol. Because statin drugs lower LDL cholesterol 30% to 50% and raise HDL cholesterol 6% to 7%, the independent clinical benefit from raising HDL cholesterol levels is difficult to determine; however, retrospective analysis of all the statin trials has shown that, among individuals on statin therapy, subjects with lower levels of HDL cholesterol had higher rates of coronary events than individuals with higher levels of HDL cholesterol. In the Lipoprotein and Coronary Atherosclerosis Study, compared with placebo, individuals on fluvastatin with HDL cholesterol levels less than 35 mg/dL had a greater reduction in angiographically measured CHD progression and more prolonged event-free survival than subjects with HDL cholesterol levels greater than 35 mg/dL.

Family History

It has been estimated that family history accounts for 65 percent of the development of CHD. About 30 percent of this is due to a single-gene that affects the way our bodies metabolize fats. For example, there is a genetic condition called familial hypercholesterolemia, that causes LDL and total cholesterol to be removed very slowly from the blood because of a deficiency of LDL receptors. In addition to abnormalities in the LDL receptor activity, defective genes may produce low HDL cholesterol levels, affect blood-clotting factors, blood pressure, and a person's insulin response. Any of these genetic conditions will be worsened if the other risk factors are present.

Family History Of Early CHD

In prospective cohort and case-control studies, family history of premature CHD is a major independent risk factor associated with increased CHD risk. CHD in a first-degree relative increases relative risk of CHD 2 to 12 times. Risk further increases with number of primary relatives affected and with younger age at onset. In contrast, the Framingham Heart Study found that family history analysis does not demonstrate sufficient incremental risk to be included in risk assessment equations. Many modifiable risk factors are also seen in people with premature CHD and with first-degree relatives with CHD, a finding suggesting that lifestyle factors are also important.

Positive family history for CHD in a first-degree relative is a major risk factor for CHD and is associated with high prevalence of modifiable risk factors. The report states that risk for CHD is higher the younger the age of onset of CHD and the greater the number of first-degree relatives with CHD. It is recommended that the presence and age of onset of CHD in all first-degree relatives be assessed.

Sex/Age

Coronary heart disease is found more commonly in men than in women. It is estimated that 1 out of 5 men and 1 out of 17 women in the United States will have symptoms of heart disease before the age of 60. This shows that men have two to three times the risk of developing CHD. After menopause, both sexes are found to be nearly equal at risk of developing heart disease. Women's blood cholesterol levels prior to menopause are generally lower than those of men of the same age.

On average, older people have more coronary atherosclerosis than younger people. Men develop CHD on average about 10 years younger than women; this difference is probably explained by the protective effect of estrogen in pre-menopausal women. Rate of CHD increase in women after menopause (whether surgical or natural). For these reasons, ATP III defines advancing age as a major independent risk factor and recommends that age 45 years or older in men and 55 years or older in women should count as a risk factor in determining an LDL cholesterol goal in primary prevention.

Obesity

There are several methods of determining overweight and obesity. A person is considered overweight if he or she is 10 to 20 percent over desirable weight or has a body mass index (BMI) above 25. Twenty percent above desirable weight, or a BMI over 30, is defined as obese.

BMI = Kg/m^2

1. Divide weight in pounds by 2.2 to convert to kilograms
   (e.g. 120 lbs. Divided by 2.2 = 55 kg)

2. Multiply height in inches by 2.5 to convert to centimeter
   (e.g. 5.2" - 62 x 2.5 = 155 centimeters

3. Divide 155 by 100 to get meters.
   155/100 = 1.6 meters

4. Square 1.6 meters = 2.56 square meters

5. BMI = 55 kg = 21
   2.56 Square meters

Fat distribution in the body plays an important role in determining susceptibility to heart disease. People who have fat distributed around the abdomen that looks like an apple have a greater risk of heart disease, high blood cholesterol, hypertension, stroke and diabetes. This type of obesity is called android. Most women have pear shaped obesity called gynoid obesity. The fat is distributed in the hips and thighs.

Abdominal obesity is determined by the ratio between the circumference of the waist and the hips. The normal range occurs when the waist measures 15 percent less than the hips. Waist measurement that exceeds hip measurement is considered a risk factor.

The risk for CVD is especially high when abdominal obesity is present (waist circumference > 102 cm (40in) in men or 88 cm (35in) in women.

Both genetics and environmental factors play a role in the development of obesity. Researchers have found that part of the mechanism that controls the number of calories we burn at rest and in digesting a meal, are genetically controlled. Environmental factors include nutritional, psychological and social influences.

Sedentary Lifestyle

Studies have shown that people who exercise regularly have fewer heart attacks. Exercise affects cardiovascular risk factors such as obesity, hypertension, and blood levels of total cholesterol, HDL, and triglyceride.

The energy expended during exercise can be either from aerobic or anaerobic metabolism. Weight lifting, sit-ups and isometrics are anaerobic exercises. These exercises use energy from stored energy sources and they burn few calories. Brisk walking, running, swimming, cycling, jumping rope or skating are aerobic exercises because oxygen is needed. The oxygen used by the body during exercise can be measured. VO_2 max (maximum oxygen uptake) refers to the greatest amount of oxygen that can be taken from the air during exercise.

The beneficial effects of regular aerobic exercise are summarized as follows:

1. Lower blood total cholesterol level
2. Higher blood HDL level
3. Decrease in heart rate (pulse rate)
4. Lower blood pressure
5. Lower body fat
6. Efficient use of blood sugar
7. Lower level of fibrinogen
8. VO_2 max increased: this enables individuals to do greater amounts of physical work.

If a person has atherosclerosis, exercise may help develop alternate (collateral) circulation that increases the heart's blood supply. Exercise is now prescribed regularly for patients with cardiovascular disease.

Before undertaking any type of exercise, it is important to have a general physical examination by a physician.

Stress

Research on heart disease and stress has focused mostly on Type A and Type B behavior patterns. Type A people are competitive, impatient and they tend to do many things at the same time. Type B people are more relaxed. Type A behavior has been associated with coronary heart disease. People whose blood pressure and heart rate increase significantly when they are faced with frustrating situations may also be more likely to develop heart disease. According to Deepak Chopra, author of "Ageless body to Oneless Mind" there is a strong connection between aging and stress hormones. Chopra suggests that meditation can play a very important healing role by going directly to the root of the stress. Studies have shown that long-term meditators and their levels of cortisol and adrenaline are lower. They have better coping mechanisms. Social bonds are also important in keeping hearts healthy. It is important to keep stress levels low by making time for pleasurable activities.

Blood Triglyceride Level

Triglyceride is the fat in the blood that the body uses to carry the fatty acids. Triglyceride from the diet is carried from the intestine on lipoproteins called chylomicrons. A number of factors can influence blood triglycerides. These include obesity, a diet high in simple carbohydrates, fat and alcohol. Several studies have shown that high blood levels of triglycerides are associated with increased risk of coronary heart disease. Desirable triglyceride levels are below 150 mg/dl.

Diet

Cholesterol: It is a natural part of such foods as lamb, pork, beef, chicken, organ meats, dairy products and eggs. A 3-ounce piece of meat, fish, or chicken has 60-90 mg of cholesterol. One egg yolk contains about 270 mg of cholesterol. Excess dietary cholesterol causes hypercholesterolemia and atherosclerosis. The degree of rise varies from person to person. Excess dietary cholesterol also contributes to high LDL-cholesterol. Total cholesterol and LDL-cholesterol levels will begin to drop 2-3 weeks after starting a cholesterol lowering diet. How much blood cholesterol levels are lowered depends on how much fat

— especially saturated fat — and how much cholesterol you were eating before starting your cholesterol-lowering diet. A cholesterol-lowering diet should be continued for life.

Saturated Fat

A high intake of saturated fats increases blood cholesterol level. Saturated fats are found primarily in animal products, particularly fatty meats and many dairy products. Coconut oil, palm kernel oil, and palm oil are also saturated.

Unsaturated oils become saturated by the process of hydrogenation, e.g. margarine. The hydrogenation process also changes the chemical structure. The new structure is called trans fatty acids.

Trans Fatty Acids

Trans-unsaturated fatty acids result when polyunsaturated fats, such as those in corn oil and soybean oil, are partially hydrogenated to produce stick margarine and shortening. In addition to use in frying fast foods, partially hydrogenated fats enhance shelf-life of bakery goods and snack foods. When substituted for energy from carbohydrates, trans fatty acids raise LDL cholesterol and the total cholesterol-to-HDL ratio, as well as possibly producing a smaller, more atherogenic LDL particle. Amounts of trans fatty acids in foods have to be listed, from January 2006.

Unsaturated Fats

There are two kinds of unsaturated fats: polyunsaturated and monosaturated. Sunflower oil, safflower oil, corn oil, and soybean oils are polyunsaturated. Olive oil and canola oil are monounsaturated. It is recommended to use more monounsaturated oils.

Fish oils are high in polyunsaturated fats and contain two unsaturated fatty acids called eicosapentaenoic acid (EPA) and docosahexaenoic acid (DAH). They are referred to as omega-3 and omega-6 fatty acids. These fats are different from animal fats. Some studies have shown beneficial effects on the profile of lipids and lipoproteins in the blood. It is recommended that you eat fish caught in cold waters at least twice a week. Fish which are excellent sources of these fatty acids include: Salmon, trout, tuna, mackerel, herring, bluefish and anchovies.

Sodium

The American Heart Association (AHA) recommends that healthy adults consume no more than 2400 mg of salt per day. This equals to 1-1/4 teaspoons.

People with hypertension may need to restrict their salt intake. It is easy to overlook sources of sodium in the diet. Besides table salt, it is found in many processed foods.

Diabetes

Diabetes is defined as fasting glucose > of 126 mg/dL which is a risk factor for CHD. Several lines of evidence support this concept. First, both persons with type I and those with type 2 diabetes have a high risk of new CHD within 10 years, which approximates the risk in patients with known CHD but no diabetes. The relative risk (but not absolute risk) in women with diabetes exceeds that in men with diabetes.

Subjects with type 1 diabetes have an increased risk for CHD; however, no study has reported whether subjects with type 1 diabetes have a CHD risk similar to that for age- and sex-matched nondiabetic subjects with clinical CHD. Such a study would be difficult to perform because subjects often develop type 1 diabetes at an early age when their contemporaries have no CHD. ATP III recommends that recent-onset type 1 diabetes is not a CHD risk equivalent and reduction of LDL cholesterol to less than 130 mg/dL is sufficient. However, an LDL cholesterol goal less than 100 mg/dL should be considered as duration of type 1 diabetes increases.

Part of the increased risk for CHD in diabetes results from the major risk factors. Management of these risk factors (blood pressure, cholesterol, and triglyceride lowering) has been shown to reduce the risk of a coronary event in patients with diabetes. The risk attributed to hyperglycemia is independent of being obese or overweight. Some studies have shown a strong association between glycemia and CHD in type 2 diabetes, whereas others have shown a weak association or no association. A trend toward benefit of controlling glucose has been shown but is not yet definitive.

Classification of diabetes as a CHD risk equivalent implies that benefit should be achieved by lowering LDL cholesterol levels. AFCAPS, a primary prevention trial, showed a 43% reduction in CHD risk in patients with diabetes on statin compared with placebo. Secondary prevention trials of statin drugs have also shown benefit in diabetes.

Atherogenic Dyslipidemia

The combination of elevated triglycerides, small LDL particles, and reduced HDL cholesterol levels is called "atherogenic dyslipidemia" and is common in people with premature CHD. Many people with type 2 diabetes have this type of dyslipidemia. There is a strong trend toward reduction in risk of CHD with treatment of atherogenic dyslipidemia. Most therapies that lower triglyceride levels or raise HDL cholesterol levels modify all components of the dyslipidemia. Weight reduction, physical activity, fibrates, and nicotinic acid specifically improve all components of atherogenic dyslipidemia. Both primary and secondary prevention trials with fibric acid derivatives, niacin, or both have shown a reduction in CHD risk.

Lipoprotein

Lipoprotein (a) [Lp(a)] is an additional protein found on LDL in some people. Several studies have found a strong association of Lp(a) and CHD, whereas other prospective studies have not shown an independent prediction. In 40 patients with Lp(a) level at or above the 90th percentile, those with an LDL cholesterol reduction greater than 10% had an event rate of 9%, compared with 36% in those with LDL cholesterol reduction less than 10%. The best correlate of baseline CVD severity was the Lp(a) level. Estrogen and niacin are the only two drugs that lower levels of Lp(a). Estrogen may be harmful, and niacin is not well tolerated. In addition, issues related to measurement have not been resolved. The immunologic assay is standardized in only a few laboratories and is not established in hospital clinical chemistry labs, so samples must be sent to specialized laboratories. Therefore, until results of randomized trials lowering Lp(a) levels are available, the best course of treatment is lowering LDL cholesterol to goal in patients with CHD. ATP III suggests that a high Lp(a) may justify a lower LDL cholesterol goal and that Lp(a) measurement be limited to people with family history of premature CHD or genetic causes of hypercholesterolemia with no other risk factors.

Homocysteine

People with inherited forms of homocysteinemia have premature vascular injury and atherosclerosis. In observational studies, elevations of homocysteine have been shown to be positively correlated with CHD risk. A randomized double blind placebo-controlled trial of 553 subjects assigned to a combined treatment (n = 272) of folic acid (1 mg/day), vitamin B-12 (cyanocobalamin, 400 μg/day), and vitamin B-6 (pyridoxine hydrochloride, 10 mg/day), or placebo (n = 281) for 6 months after percutaneous transluminal coronary angioplasty (PTCA) showed that adverse cardiovascular endpoints were significantly reduced in subjects on folic acid. In an open-label trial, 593 patients with CHD were randomized to 0.5 mg folic acid or control; all subjects were on statins. At mean follow-up of 24 months, homocysteine levels were lowered 18% (from 12 to 9.4 mg/dL); however, all-cause mortality and a composite of vascular events were not significantly different in subjects on folic acid compared with the control group (10.3% vs 9.6%, respectively; relative risk: 1./05; 95% confidence interval: 0.63.

The American Heart Association recommends supplemental folic acid to patients with high homocysteine level. ATP III does not recommend routine measurement of homocysteine as part of assessment to modify LDL cholesterol levels because of uncertainty about the strength of relation with CHD. Measurement is an option for cases with a strong family history of premature CHD. If a person is otherwise at low risk, ATP III recommends treating with B vitamins and folic acid because treatment is safe and inexpensive. Breakfast cereals, broccoli, oranges, flour, and multivitamins have high amounts of folic acid.

C-Reactive Protein (CRP)

Recent articles indicate that serum levels of CRP are predictive of coronary events. Smoking is associated with increased CRP levels. Obesity and metabolic syndrome are also commonly accompanied by increases in CRP, so there is likely a relationship between metabolic factors and inflammation.

High-sensitivity (hs)-CRP may have independent predictive power beyond lipid risk factors. A randomized trial is currently under way to determine whether lowering CRP with rosuvastatin decreases CHD events in primary prevention. Statin drugs and aspirin lower CRP, and in secondary prevention both should be prescribed.

CHAPTER 2

METABOLIC SYNDROME

Metabolic syndrome (MES) has been called by many names: syndrome X, insulin resistance syndrome, and the multiple metabolic syndrome. It consists of a cluster of risk factors responsible for much of the cardiovascular disease (CVD) morbidity among overweight and obese patients and those with type 2 diabetes mellitus. The National Cholesterol Education Program (NCEP) Adult Treatment Panel III report (ATP III) has identified MES as an independent risk factor for CVD and considers it an indication for intensive lifestyle modification. The major characteristics of MES include insulin resistance (IR), abdominal obesity, elevated blood pressure, and lipid abnormalities: elevated triglycerides and low HDL cholesterol levels. MES is also associated with a proinflammatory, prothrombotic state that may include elevated CRP, endothelial dysfunction, increased platelet aggregation, elevated uric acid levels, microalbuminuria, and a shift toward small dense LDL particles. IR has been implicated in the polycystic ovarian syndrome and nonalcoholic steatohepatitis (NASH).

Based on data from the Third National Health and Nutrition Examination Survey, it is estimated that 22% to 24% of the adult US population has MES. Among comparable age groups, prevalence of MES in the United States is highest in Mexican Americans and lowest in African Americans. The prevalence of MES increases with age and with increasing body weight. Given the aging American population and the current epidemic of overweight and obesity, MES is likely to soon overtake cigarette smoking as the primary contributor to risk of CVD.

Although the etiology of MES has not been definitively established, two theories have been proposed. Abdominal obesity, independent of body mass index (BMI), plays a role in both theories. One hypothesis assumes that the primary lesion is IR, which correlates with abdominal fat measured by waist circumference or waist-to-hip ratio. Supporting this theory, data from the Nurses' Health Study showed a threefold increased risk of CVD in women with a waist circumference above 38 inches (after adjusting for age and other known risk factors). The link between IR and CVD is probably mediated by oxidative stress, which produces endothelial cell dysfunction, promoting vascular damage and atheroma formation. A second hypothesis places importance on hormonal changes, principally elevated serum cortisol levels.

A routine medical and family history helps to identify patients at risk for MES. Questions in the review of systems about recent or past weight changes and efforts to gain or lose weight may provide important information. A diet and physical history, including both occupational and leisure-time physical activity, should be part of the routine patient evaluation. Have patients estimate how many hours a day they are sedentary (watching TV or sitting at a desk). Questions about typical food intake and efforts to reduce dietary fat or other specific dietary changes help to provide a clue to patients' awareness of CVD risk and help to estimate their readiness to change lifestyle habits.

Height and weight, as well as blood pressure and waist circumference, should be measured as part of the physical examination. Waist circumference is measured just above the iliac crest. Waist circumference appears to be a better predictor of CVD risk than waist-to-hip ratio. BMI should be assessed to classify patients as underweight, normal weight, overweight, or obese.

Clinicians should obtain a fasting glucose level and a fasting lipid profile on patients suspected of having MES. Fasting insulin and glucose levels can be measured to establish a diagnosis of IR. However, these levels are not as accurate as a euglycemic clamp, which is used in research studies but is impractical in the clinical setting. Fasting blood glucose or fasting insulin levels are both good indication of IR, but measuring insulin levels is probably not necessary in most situations. It is not necessary to measure apolipoprotein B levels if LDL is normal because low HDL cholesterol and high triglyceride (TG) levels are predictive of small dense LDL particles, which raise apo B level. Although there is no consensus on how to treat elevated CRP levels, the American Heart Association (AHA) recommends measuring CRP in high-risk patients. Baseline uric acid levels and routine liver function tests, such as alanine aminotransferase (ALT), aspartate aminotransferase (AST), and gamma-glutamyltranspeptidase (GTP) levels, screen for NASH, but fatty liver can be present even in the absence of elevated liver function tests.

A word of caution in interpreting the results of laboratory studies: the lack of any individual component of the syndrome does not mean a patient is free of risk. Many patients who do not meet the full criteria of MES have an increased risk of CVD from the component of the syndrome they do have.

Assessment of the Patient

ATP III outlines ten steps to assess CHD risk in patients, determine their LDL cholesterol goals, and establish treatment and follow-up plans.

1. Lipid Measurements
   ATP III guidelines recommend that a 9- to 12-hour fasting complete lipid profile be determined in adults age 20 and older every 5 years. This profile should include total cholesterol, HDL, LDL, and triglyceride levels. Glucose levels should also be measured to assess for the presence of diabetes or metabolic syndrome. In patients with hyperlipidemia, it is important to rule out secondary causes of high cholesterol because such causes may necessitate treatment other than lipid-lowering drugs. Major causes include hypothyroidism, diabetes, multiple myeloma, and obstructive liver disease. Laboratory values that are important in assessing these secondary causes include thyroid stimulating hormone, fasting glucose, serum and urine protein electrophoresis, aspartate aminotransferase (AST), alanine aminotransferase (ALT), and alkaline phosphatase.

2. Identify Clinical CHD or Risk Equivalent
   Taking a careful history for the presence of angina pectoris, history of MI, diabetes, transient ischemic attack, or pain in the calves or thighs with exercise (claudication) is most important in determining whether clinical atherosclerosis is present. If any of these are present, the LDL cholesterol goal is less than 100 mg/dL.

3. Determine Presence of Major Risk Factors
   (Other than LDL Cholesterol)
   When determining a patient's LDL cholesterol goal, the number of major risk factors – cigarette smoking, hypertension, low HDL cholesterol level, family history of premature CHD, and age – should be counted. Smoking, family history, and age can be obtained from the history. If HDL cholesterol is greater than 60 mg/dL (measured as in step 1), one risk factor is subtracted. During the physical exam, blood pressure, height, weight, and waist circumference should be measured and BMI calculated.

   Blood pressure should be measured using the auscultatory method with a properly calibrated and validated cuff that encircles at least 80% of the arm. Patients should be seated quietly in a chair (rather than on an exam table) for at least 5 minutes with feet on the floor and arm supported at heart level. At least two measurements should be made.

Routine laboratory test recommended for the evaluation of hypertension include urinalysis, blood glucose, hematocrit, serum potassium, creatinine (or estimated glomerular filtration rate), calcium, and electrocardiogram. The JNC 7 guidelines state that urinary albumin excretion is option; however, it should be performed in patients with diabetes. Ninety percent of cases of hypertension result from essential hypertension where no identifiable cause is apparent. If blood pressure control is not achieved, identifiable causes of hypertension should be considered. Causes include sleep apnea, drugs (nonsteroidal anti-inflammatory drugs, cyclooxygenase 2 inhibitors, cocaine, amphetamines, decongestants, anorectics, oral contraceptives, cyclosporine and tacrolimun, erythropoietin, licorice, and over-the-counter dietary supplements [ephedra, ma haung, and bitter orange]), chronic kidney disease, primary aldosteronism, renovascular disease, chronic steroid therapy of cushing syndrome, pheochromocytoma, aortic coarctation, and thyroid or parathyroid disease.

Metabolic syndrome should also be assessed at the initial visit. Initial treatment is implementing Therapeutic Lifestyle Changes (TLC) as described in ATP III. Because weight loss can take time, it is important to counsel the patient as early as possible to increase physical activity and change diet in an attempt to lose weight. Small, realistic weight loss goals are important. Weight loss of 5% to 10% of body weight has been shown to be beneficial. Because the presence of abdominal obesity is more highly correlated with high triglycerides, low HDL cholesterol levels, increased blood pressure, and elevated fasting glucose than is BMI, ATP III recommends use of waist circumference measurement to identify the body weight component of metabolic syndrome.

4-5. Determine Risk Category and Establish LDL Cholesterol Goal

Determining a patient's CHD risk category is necessary to identify the LDL cholesterol goal. Calculation of a 10-year CHD risk using the Framingham risk scores allows more precise differentiation of an appropriate LDL cholesterol goal.

- For people with low risk (< 2 risk factors), the 10-year risk assessment is not needed.
- For people with two or more risk factors, the 10-year risk assessment yields one of three levels of 10-year risk: (a) less than 10%; (b) 10% to 20%; or (c) greater than 20%.

For a 10-year risk less than 10%, the LDL cholesterol threshold at which to start drug therapy is greater than 160 mg/dL. For a 10-year risk of 10% to 20%, ATP III indicates drug therapy when LDL cholesterol is greater than 130 mg/dL. However, a July 2004 update to ATP III includes drug therapy as an option for LDL cholesterol between 100 and 129 mg/dL. Those with a risk greater than 20-% are placed in the same category as subjects with established CHD, and the LDL cholesterol goal is less than 100 mg/dL according to ATP III and less than 70 mg/dL according to the ATP III update.

6. Initiate TLC if LDL Cholesterol is Above Goal
   Once a patient's risk category is determined and the LDL cholesterol goal is established, the need for TLC or drug consideration is assessed. If the patient's current LDL cholesterol level is above the goal level, then TLC therapy is initiated. The TLC diet consists of less than 7% of energy from saturated fat and less than 200 mg of cholesterol per day, increased soluble (viscous) fiber (10 to 25 g/day), and plant stanol or sterols (2 g/day) to enhance LDL lowering. Weight management is encouraged both through diet and increased physical activity.

7. Consider Adding Drug Therapy If LDL Cholesterol Exceeds Threshold Levels
   Drug therapy is often started simultaneously with TLC for patients with CHD, diabetes, and CHD risk equivalents. After at lease 3 months of TLC, if LDL cholesterol does not reach the level, consider adding drug therapy to TLC. TLC therapy should complement drug therapy and should be continually encouraged. Common drug classes are the statins, bile acid sequestrants, nicotinic acid, and fibric acids. One class may be sufficient, but drugs can be combined if necessary to reach goal.

8. Identify Metabolic Syndrome and Treat, If Present, After 3 Months of TLC
   Identifying and treating metabolic syndrome is important because this condition can lead to diabetes. The underlying causes of metabolic syndrome (obesity, physical inactivity, and insulin resistance) are most simply and effectively treated by intensifying weight management and increasing physical activity.

   After 3 months of TLC, the lipid and nonlipid risk factors should also be treated if they persist despite the lifestyle therapies. Hypertension should be treated with antihypertensives, the prothrombotic state should be treated with aspirin and elevated triglyceride or low HDL cholesterol levels should be treated.

9. Treat Elevated Triglyceride Levels

Causes of elevated triglyceride levels include being overweight or obese, physical inactivity, cigarette smoking, excess alcohol intake, very high (> 60%) carbohydrate diets, other diseases (type 2 diabetes, chronic renal failure, nephrotic syndrome), some drugs (corticosteroids, protease inhibitors for human immunodeficiency virus, beta-adrenergic blocking agents, estrogen), and genetic factors. Weight management can be intensified and physical activity increased to lower triglyceride levels.

If triglyceride levels are still 200 mg/dL or higher after the LDL cholesterol goal is met, the secondary goal for non-HDL cholesterol (total cholesterol minus HDL cholesterol) is set 30 mg/dL higher than the LDL cholesterol goal. If triglyceride levels are 200 to 499 mg/dL after the LDL cholesterol goal is reached, intensify therapy with an LDL cholesterol-lowering drug or add nicotine acid or fibrate to lower VLDL. Improving blood glucose management in patients with elevated glucose can also improve triglyceride levels.

If triglyceride levels are 500 mg/dL or higher, triglycerides are lowered first to prevent pancreatitis. The patient should be put on a very-low-fat diet (< 15% of energy from fat) and should be advised on weight management and physical activity and to abstain from alcohol ingestion. Fibrate or nicotinic acid may be necessary. When triglycerides are less than 500 mg/dL, consider whether LDL cholesterol-lowering therapy is necessary.

10. Treat Low HDL Cholesterol Levels (<40 mg/dL)

First, reach the LDL cholesterol goal. Once the LDL cholesterol goal is reached, if the HDL cholesterol level is less than 40 mg/dL, weight management and physical activity should be increased. Potentially reversible causes of low HDL cholesterol levels include high triglyceride levels, cigarette smoking, type 2 diabetes, being overweight or obese, physical inactivity, very high carbohydrate intake (> 60%), and drugs such as beta-blockers, anabolic steriods, and progestational agents. Hygienic measures to raise HDL cholesterol levels include modifying the underlying cause through diet and weight loss in the overweight and obese, increased physical activity in the sedentary, and smoking cessation. These measures should be instituted first to raise HDL cholesterol levels in both primary and secondary prevention.

If the triglyceride level is 200 to 499 mg/dL, achieve the non-HDL cholesterol goal. If the triglyceride levels are less than 200 mg/dL (isolated low HDL cholesterol) in CHD or CHD equivalent, nicotinic acid or fibrate should be considered.

TREATMENT STRATEGIES

To date, no randomized controlled trials aimed specifically at treating MES have been published. By aggressively managing the individual components of the syndrome, the goal is to prevent or delay the onset of diabetes, hypertension, and CVD. All patients diagnosed with MES should be encouraged to attempt to change their diet and exercise habits as primary therapy. Weight loss improves all aspects of MES and reduces all-cause morbidity and CVD mortality. Although many patients find weight loss difficult to achieve, dietary changes can lower blood pressure and improve lipid levels. Increasing exercise can improve insulin sensitivity even in the absence of weight loss.

Physical Activity

As an insulin-sensitive tissue, skeletal muscle is a primary target for affecting IR. Physical training has been shown to reduce skeletal muscle lipid levels and IR for individuals across the BMI range. Exercise training increases the muscle's ability to take up and oxidize free fatty acids. Exercise has been shown to lower systolic blood pressure by an average of 4 to 9 mm Hg in patients with elevated blood pressure. Regular exercise reverses the age-related decline in insulin sensitivity independent of weight loss or increases in maximum oxygen consumption (VO_{2max}). The impact of exercise on insulin sensitivity is evident for 24 to 48 hours and disappears within 3 to 5 days. Thus, regular physical activity should be a part of any effort to reverse the effect of IR.

Exercise alone has not been shown to reduce body weight; thus, the importance of exercise for weight loss is unclear. Exercise, however, is the best predictor of weight-loss maintenance and has been shown to improve hemoglobin Alc in patients who have not lost weight. In a meta-analysis of studies published on the impact of exercise in patients with type 2 diabetes, it has been concluded that exercise should be considered a desirable endpoint and not just a means to achieve weight loss.

The Institute of Medicine's Dietary Reference Intakes for Energy recommends 1 hour of physical activity daily for health maintenance. This recommendation has been made to prevent continued weight gain in the population. The greatest health benefits from an increase in physical activity occur when sedentary individuals incorporate moderate-intensity exercise as part of their lifestyle.

Low-intensity exercise can have a significant impact on cardiorespiratory fitness. It is easier to get patients to comply with less-intensive and less-frequent exercise regimens. It is important to encourage patients to find their own comfort level for physical activity rather than assigning them a specific task. The goal is to help patients find a level of activity that they can accomplish over the long term. A combination of resistance and aerobic exercise is advised, but any activity is better than none, and patients who have been sedentary need to start slowly and increase duration and intensity gradually. Patients should be encouraged to do some type of aerobic and resistance exercise on alternating days. Low-weight dumbbells, stretchy bands, or even 16-ounce food cans provide the needed resistance. Circuit-type resistance training machines, if available, maximize the impact of muscle strengthening. The ultimate goal may be 1 hour of daily physical activity (walking or any combination of lifestyle activities), but in working up to that goal, patients should start with 1 to 2 days per week for 5 to 10 minutes at 50% of maximal heart rate and increase gradually.

DIET PRESCRIPTION

The first step in developing a diet prescription is the evaluation of the patient's current diet. This can be done during the course of the history with a few pertinent questions. The primary emphasis of the diet should focus on reducing CVD risk. If the patient has elevated LDL cholesterol, recommend a low-fat moderate-carbohydrate diet (total fat 25% to 35% of energy, saturated fat less than 7%, with carbohydrate as 45% to 60% of energy). Both epidemiologic data and clinical trial results have shown this diet to be effective in reducing LDL cholesterol and lowering CVD risk.

Although the NCEP recommends that carbohydrates comprise the major source of energy (50% to 60% of total energy), patients need to be aware of both the quantity and quality of their carbohydrate intake because excessive consumption of carbohydrates may increase TG levels while depressing HDL cholesterol levels.

According to the AHA and ATP III, the intake of added sugars should be minimized, while the intake of whole grains that are higher in fiber should be increased. The glycemic index (GI) categorizes or ranks carbohydrate-containing foods according to the extent to which they raise blood glucose levels after eating. Initial studies analyzed the blood glucose response using 50 g of pure glucose compared with 50 g of a carbohydrate-containing food. However, the standard to which carbohydrate foods are now compared has been changed to white bread. Diets tailored to lower the GI have been shown in small studies to reduce TG levels and raise HDL cholesterol levels. A recent observational study further supports a high-fiber, low-GI diet for patients at risk for MES. Because many variables affect the blood glucose response of a particular carbohydrate-containing food, some controversy exists concerning the usefulness of GI as a tool in the nutrition management of MES, diabetes, or hyperlipidemia.

Fiber. ATP III recommends the inclusion of 20 to 30 g/day of dietary fiber, 10 ro 25 g/day of which should come from soluble or viscous fiber. In the United States the average fiber intake is only 15 g//day. Oatmeal, beans, citrus fruits, split peas, and broccoli are some of the best sources of soluble fiber, with approximately 2 to 4 g per serving. Foods that contain dietary fiber often take longer to eat and may increase satiety by delaying gastric emptying, which may assist in glucose handling and weight management. Observational studies have also reported that diets high in fiber can even delay the onset of diabetes. The quality and quantity of carbohydrate intake can easily be assessed by asking patients four simple questions:

Key Nutrition History Questions

- Drinks During The Day? How Many Glasses?
- Type of Snacks and Desserts?
- Fats and Oils?
- Sodium and Calcium Intake
- Salt Use
- Diary Products

Finally, because individuals respond differently to dietary changes, laboratory tests should be monitored. If patients develop hypertriglyceridemia or fail to show improvements in serum lipid levels, then fiber intake can be increased (with a goal of 25 to 35 g/day) or carbohydrate intake can be reduced and replaced with monounsaturated fatty acid. This diet should still emphasize high-fiber, lower GI foods. The long-term effects of low-carbohydrate diets have not been adequately studied, but short term, these diets have been shown to lower TGs, raise HDL cholesterol, and reduce body weight. If patients choose a low-carbohydrate diet plan, advise them to select lean meats and MUFAs and to limit saturated fats.

Pharmacotherapy

After lifestyle adjustment has been addressed, the treatment of MES focuses on treating any cardiovascular or diabetes risk factors the patient may have.

ATP III guidelines classify MES as a secondary therapeutic target after the initial treatment of any LDL cholesterol abnormalities. Treatment of LDL cholesterol with statins has proven to be effective in reducing cardiovascular events in patients with diabetes, a population with a high proportion of patients with MES. The Heart Protection Study, a placebo-controlled, randomized trial, included a subpopulation of nearly 6,000 patients with diabetes. This study showed that in a high-risk population including those with diabetes, simvastatin not only lowered LDL cholesterol levels but significantly reduced vascular events.

For patients with hypertriglyceridemia, fibrates such as gemfibrozil or fenofibrate are peroxisome proliferator-activated receptor (PPAR)-alpha agonists, which act primarily by increasing fatty-acid oxidation and thus lead to reductions in TG synthesis and very-low-density lipoprotein (VLDL) secretion. Moreover, fibrates increase the expression of apo A-I, consequently leading to a beneficial increase in HDL cholesterol level. In the veteran Affairs High-Density Lipoprotein Intervention Study (VA-HIT), gemfibrozil treatment was associated with a 35% decrease in relative risk for a combined cardiovascular end point among patients with diabetes.

Although the use of niacin was previously contraindicated in patients with IR because it may increase levels of blood glucose and aggravate IR, recent trials indicate a potential role for niacin therapy in patients with MES. A report on the Arterial Disease Multiple Intervention Trial showed an association between niacin therapy and decreased TG levels, as well as increased HDL cholesterol, in patients with diabetes. And although this study did confirm that niacin raises blood glucose in people both with and without diabetes, the levels of glycated hemoglobin did not change in the patients with diabetes or IR, although care must be taken to monitor glucose levels.

Antihypertensive agents should be included when blood pressure needs to be lowered. Beta-blocker therapy had been withheld from patients with either diabetes or IR because of its ability to mask hypoglycemic symptoms. However, beta-blockers can significantly reduce cardiovascular mortality among patients with diabetes and hypertension and should consequently receive consideration. Also, there is compelling evidence not only that treatment of hypertension with angiotensin-converting enzyme inhibitors (ACE inhibitors) is beneficial for its effect on lowering blood pressure, but that it may also prove to reduce the risk of other complications of diabetes such as nephropathy and CVD.

PREVENTION

The US Prevention Services Task Force recommends intensive behavior and dietary counseling for adult patients with known risk factors for CVD. The Diabetes Prevention Program demonstrated that vigorous lifestyle intervention could prevent the onset of diabetes by more than 50% (from 11% to 4.8%).

Patients randomized to the control, metformin, or lifestyle interventions all ate fewer total calories. The control and metformin groups reduced their daily energy intake by 250 and 300 kcal, respectively, whereas the lifestyle group reduced their intake by 400 kcal. Patients initially consumed 35% of their energy from fat; with dietary instruction, they reduced their fat intake by 6%. Although the many individual counseling sessions provided to each patient during 2 to 3 years is clearly beyond what physician practices can offer as part of routine care, efforts are being made to educate family physicians on how to conduct brief counseling sessions for patients with MES.

CHAPTER 3

MEDICAL NUTRITION THERAPY GUIDELINES (ATP III GUIDELINES)

After determining a patient's risk category, decision should be made regarding initiation of Medical Nutrition Therapy (MNT). The following recommendations are noted:

1. Nutrients that raise LDL cholesterol should be minimized.
   - Reduce dietary saturated fat to less than 7% of total energy.
   - Reduce dietary cholesterol to less than 200 mg/day.
   - Total dietary fat should be in the range of 25% to 35% of total energy.

2. Therapeutic options may be added for further lowering of LDL cholesterol
   - Plant stanols and sterols can be added (2 g/day).
   - Viscous fiber may be increased to 10 to 25 g/day
   - Total energy intake should be adjusted to maintain desirable body weight and prevent weight gain.

3. Physical activity should include moderate exercise to expend 200 or more kcal/day.

The macronutrient distribution should be approximately 15% of energy from protein, 50% to 60% of energy from carbohydrate, and 25% to 35% of energy from fat. From a macronutrient perspective, nutrition recommendations to reduce the risk of CHD include the following:

1. Limit intake of cholesterol-raising saturated fat and trans fat. Replace with monounsaturated fat and, to some extent, polyunsaturated fat.
2. Emphasize carbohydrate intake from whole grains, fruits, and vegetables to provide complex carbohydrate, dietary fiber, vitamins, and other antioxidants.
3. Choose protein from sources that limit saturated fat and can provide n-3 fatty acids, isoflavones, and monounsaturated fats.

The AHA, ATP III, and the American Dietetic Association's MNT Evidence-Based Guide provide guidelines for nutrition and heart disease. AHA provides food-based guidance for the public to prevent CHD. The other two sets of guidelines are more specific, nutrient-based guidelines designed for the primary and secondary prevention of CHD events in patients with risk factors for CHD.

Saturated Fatty Acids

Reducing and maintaining low dietary saturated fat is a major step toward optimizing the serum lipids to prevent CHD and reduce risk. Dietary saturated fatty acids, as contrasted with unsaturated fatty acids, decrease synthesis and activation of receptors, raising serum LDL cholesterol and providing an environment conducive to atherogenesis. A 1% increase in energy from saturated fat raises serum LDL cholesterol approximately 2%.

The degree to which LDL cholesterol can be lowered can vary depending upon initial lipid levels and concomitant dietary changes, such as further restriction of dietary cholesterol or addition of soluble fiber. A diet with 30% energy from total fat, less than 10% energy from saturated fat, and less than 300 mg cholesterol/day lowered LDL cholesterol by 12%, and by 16% with further reduction of saturated fat and cholesterol. A recent clinical trial restricting energy from saturated fat to 7% and cholesterol to less than 200 mg lowered LDL cholesterol by 11%. Large, randomized clinical trials of a similar diet reported LDL cholesterol was lowered by 11% and 8%.

How does the goal of lowering saturated fat to less than 7% of energy compared with the typical American diet? Based on the Continuing Survey of Food Intakes by Individuals (CSFII), Americans' saturated fat intake has decreased from 12.6% of energy in 1989-1991 to 11.3% in 1994-1996. National data are not yet available to adequately assess whether the popularity of low-carbohydrate diets has altered the trend in lowering saturated fat intake.

Saturated fat in the American diet is primarily from four specific fatty acids (lauric, myristic, palmitic, and stearic). A recent meta-analysis concluded lauric acid has the greatest LDL-raising effect, followed by myristic and then palmitic acids. Stearic acid lowers LDL cholesterol; however, both lauric and stearic acids lower the total cholesterol-to-HDL ratio, pointing to myristic and palmitic acids as the major dietary villains among fatty acids.

Trans Fatty Acids

Several types of evidence indicate the detrimental effects of trans fatty acids. A meta-analysis of eight controlled clinical trials has allowed prediction of the effect of particular fats on total cholesterol-to-HDL cholesterol. Although the prediction indicates coconut and palm kernel as slightly beneficial using the total cholesterol-to-HDL cholesterol ratio, these saturated fats are not encouraged based on their effect on LDL cholesterol. Of more significance is the depiction of how trans fatty acid sources such as stick margarine and shortening raise the total cholesterol-to-HDL cholesterol ratio. One recent clinical trial provided six variations of diets to 50 normocholesterolemic men in a crossover design. When trans fatty acids replaced 8% of energy from carbohydrates, LDL cholesterol was raised 10%. In another study, metabolic diets using a spectrum of fat sources (butter, soybean oil, semiliquid margarine, shortening, or stick margarine) were provided a mildly hypercholesterolemic men and women older than 50 years. LDL cholesterol levels were highest when subjects were on the diet using butter and were reduced proportionately in diets using products with fewer or no trans fatty acids. LDL cholesterol levels were 5% lower then subjects used stick margarine, 9% lower when subjects used tub margarine, and 12% lower when subjects used soybean oil. Trans fatty acids did not alter other risk factors such as blood pressure and CRP.

About one fourth of the trans fatty acids originates naturally in foods such as milk and meat, whereas the majority of trans fatty acids are introduced into the diet through hydrogenated vegetable oils. The major sources of trans fatty acids in the diets of pregnancy Canadian women were baked good (33% of trans fatty acid intake), fast food (12%), breads (10%), snacks (10%), and margarine or shortening (8%). An analysis performed for Consumer Reports provides a comparison of the saturated and trans fatty acid content of common snack foods.

A Food and Drug Administration (FDA) regulation requires that manufacturers specify grams of trans fatty acids per serving on the Nutrition Facts label on packaged foods beginning January 1, 2006. This requirement will likely prompt the food industry to use healthier fats in food preparation, as already observed when a major snack food producer switched to liquid oils and now list 0 g trans fatty acids on food labels. Based on the amount of products sold across the United States, this change is expected to lower the trans fat intake of Americans by an average of 0.2 g/day.

Monounsaturated Fatty Acids

When saturated and trans fatty acids are limited in the diet, carbohydrate or unsaturated fat can replace the unhealthy fat, providing an equivalent amount of energy. Monounsaturated fatty acids occur naturally in the *cis* form in olive oil, canola oil, avocado, olives, pecans, peanuts, and other nuts. Several guidelines allow for individualization of macronutrient proportions to increase energy from monounsaturated fat. Benefit of replacing saturated fat with monounsaturated fat is because the latter lowered LDL cholesterol levels without lowering HDL cholesterol levels. When substituted for carbohydrate, monounsaturated fat also reduces serum triglyceride levels.

Decreasing the proportion of saturated to monounsaturated fat in the diet from 2:1 to 1:2, LDL cholesterol levels decreased by almost 20% without a significant change in HDL or trigluceride levels. Although some studies suggest a benefit of liberal intake of monounsaturated fats, there are no large intervention trials testing the benefit of a higher monounsaturated fat intake on CHD events as endpoints.

The monounsaturated fat content of many nuts is one of the reasons for increasing attention to the benefit of nuts. In addition, they are a natural source of vitamin E and dietary fiber. A study of pecan intake by normolipidemic individuals reported significantly lower cholesterol in the small group randomized to include 2 ounces of pecans in the daily diet.

Polyunsaturated Fatty Acids: N-3 and N-6

Polyunsaturated fatty acids, those containing more than one double bond, can be subdivided into n-3 and n-6 fatty acids. In n-3 fatty acids, the first double bond occurs after the third carbon from the methy end of the compound; in n-6 the first double bond occurs after the sixth carbon. Of the two essential fatty acids, linoleic and linolenic, linoleic is the n-6 polyunsaturated fatty acid found in vegetable oils, such as corn, safflower, and sunflower oils. Alpha-linolenic is the n-3 polyunsaturated fatty acid, found primarily in flaxseed oil, but also present in canola, soybean, and mustard seed oil. Substitution of saturated fat with polyunsaturated fat lowers LDL cholesterol levels. N-3 fatty acids serve as precursors for eicosanoids, producing an environment that reduces platelet aggregation as well as possibly reducing inflammation. This benefit can arise from directly consuming the long-chain fish oils or ingesting the 18-carbon-alpha-linolenic acid that is elongated and desaturated within the body. Clinical trials in several countries from the 1960s and 1970s that reduced saturated fat and increased polyunsaturated fat in the diet have shown significant reduction in CHD when polyunsaturated fat was increased along with reducing dietary saturated fat.

Views of the benefits of monounsaturated vs polyunsaturated fats have fluctuated during recent years. However, the current interpretation of research findings is that dietary saturated and trans fatty acids should be limited, and naturally occurring *cis*-monounsaturated and polyunsaturated fats are similarly heart healthy.

Dietary Cholesterol

Metabolic diet studies indicate that dietary cholesterol increases total serum cholesterol approximately 10 mg/dL for every 100 mg of dietary cholesterol consumed per 1,000 kcal. By controlling saturated fat intake, dietary cholesterol intake usually decreases. Egg yolks, the most common source of dietary cholesterol, should be limited. Studies have shown that the dietary cholesterol in one egg yolk per day significantly worsened the total cholesterol-to-HDL cholesterol ratio. In another study, it has been reported that a nonsignificant increase in LDL cholesterol when two eggs per day were added to the diets of patients with hypercholesterolemia; however, the increase was significant among subjects with both elevated cholesterol and triglyceride levels.

DIETARY RECOMMENDATIONS FOR TOTAL FAT

In addition to ensuring a good fat quality by the inclusion of unsaturated rather than saturated fat, one needs to address the optimum proportion of total fat in the diet. Until recently, the long-standing dietary recommendation for total fat was that it be no more than 30% of total energy. Because no lower limit was set, questions were raised in clinical practice about what the specific level of total fat should be. Routinely, 30% became the target value; however, this goal was translated broadly and some health professionals advocated very-low-fat (<15% to 20% of energy) diets.

Recently, new dietary recommendations include ranges for total fat intake. ATP III recommends 25% to 35% of energy from fat, and the DRI report on macronutrients recommends 20% to 35% of energy from fat. The lower limit is justified to achieve adherence because a diet even lower in total fat is difficult for most individuals living in developed countries to follow. The higher limit takes into consideration the potential for adverse effects on risk factors for CHD. Higher fat diets are moderately hypercaloric compared with lower fat diets in ad libitum condition The new ranges in total fat intake still raise questions about the ideal level of dietary fat for individuals. Clinical judgement must be applied. Irrespective of level of total fat recommended, saturated fat should be kept low (< 7% of energy) to achieve and maintain desirable total and LDL cholesterol levels. Guidance is needed regarding the appropriate level of dietary fat to prescribe for practitioners who deal with many different patient profiles. Total fat affects important lipid risk factors beyond LDL cholesterol, notably, triglycerides, HDL cholesterol, non-HDL cholesterol, the ratios of total cholesterol-to-HDL cholesterol and LDL cholesterol-to-HDL cholesterol, and small, dense LDL particles. Total fat also affects postprandial plasma glucose and insulin levels, especially in individuals with type 2 diabetes. Elevated levels of postprandial plasma glucose and insulin over time may increase risk of diabetes and CHD. The preferred total fat intake is based on these parameters to reduce CHD risk. Control of energy intake must also be achieved to promote a healthy body weight and avoid overweight and obesity.

How Total Fat Affects CHD Risk

ATP III considers a low HDL cholesterol level (< 40 mg/dL) to be a major risk factor for CHD. Conversely, a high HDL cholesterol level (>60 mg/dL) is considered to be a negative risk factor for CHD; that is, it removes one risk factor from the total count of risk factors present. Elevated triglycerides, defined as 150 mg/dL or higher, are associated with an increased risk for CHD; ATP III recommends that elevated serum triglycerides be targeted for reduction initially using a lifestyle approach. Non-HDL cholesterol (the sum of very-low-density lipoprotein [VLDL] and LDL cholesterol) is highly predictive of CHD risk, especially in persons with high triglyceride levels (> 200 mg/dL).

The ratios of total cholesterol-to-HDL cholesterol and LDL cholesterol-to-HDL cholesterol are used frequently to assess CHD risk. Changes in these ratios reflect corresponding alterations in the component lipoproteins that comprise the ratio. Small, dense LDL particles are an emerging risk factor for CHD. As compared with the larger, more buoyant particles, these smaller, dense LDL particles have been associated with a greater risk of myocardial infarction, ischemic heart disease, and various types of CHD. Frequently, patients with elevated triglycerides or low HDL cholesterol or both have an accompanying elevation in small LDL particles. This combination of lipid risk factors is termed "atherogenic dyslipidemia." This profile frequently accompanies metabolic syndrome, which increases CHD risk. Metabolic syndrome consists of the following components: atherogenic dyslipidemia, elevated blood pressure, glucose intolerance, a prothrombotic state, and a proinflammatory state. The ATP III report proposes a simple clinical scheme to allow for a clinical diagnosis. According to this scheme, if a person has three of the following five characteristics, this person can be said to have metabolic syndrome:

1. Abdominal obesity (waist circumference > 40 inches in men; > 35 inches in women)
2. Triglyceride levels of 150 mg/dL or more
3. HDL cholesterol levels lower than 40 mg/dL in men, lower than 50 mg/dL in women
4. Blood pressure of 130/85 mm Hg or higher
5. Fasting glucose levels of 110 mg/dL or more (redefined as > 100 mg/dL by the American Diabetes Association in 2003)

A high postprandial glucose response might lead to the accumulation of glycated products or advanced glycation end products that promote atherogenesis. There is evidence that total fat can affect these CHD risk factors. As a result, using these risk factors can help establish what the fat level should be to reduce CHD risk beyond that attained by lowering LDL cholesterol.

Effects on Triglycerides

Serum triglycerides rise when the percentage of energy from dietary fat is decreased as the percentage of energy from carbohydrate is increased. Increasing total fat at the expense of carbohydrate is associated with small decreases in triglycerides. Based on regression analysis, every 5% decrease in total fat is predicted to increase triglycerides by 6%. Emerging evidence further indicates that dietary fiber, particularly soluble fiber, may play a role in preventing the hypertriglyceridemic response that occurs when dietary fat is reduced.

Using data from the Dietary Approaches to Stop Hypertension (DASH) Study, it has been reported that a diet providing 28% total fat and 7% saturated fat, as well as high dietary fiber (30 g/day), significantly lowered total and LDL cholesterol levels without altering triglycerides compared with a control diet (37% total fat, 14% saturated fat, 11 g/day fiber). Triglycerides also were unchanged in a study comparing a typical Western diet (39% total fat, 15% saturated fat, 10 g fiber/1,000 kcal) to a TLC diet (28% total fat, 7% saturated fat, 16 g fiber/1,000 kcal) in subjects with moderate hypercholesterolemia. It was found that a high-fiber diet (50 g/day) significantly reduced triglycerides by 10.2% below that of a diet containing 24 g/day of dietary fiber in subjects with type 2 diabetes mellitus. Both diets contained 30% of energy from total fat and 7% from saturated fat. Inclusion of high-fiber foods may prevent an increase and possibly decrease triglycerides in individuals consuming diets reduced in total fat (ie, high in carbohydrate) compared with a reduced fat diet that is low in dietary fiber. In most patients, increasing fiber-rich foods while reducing total fat can optimize the lipid profile. Higher total fat may be appropriate for some patients to decrease triglyceride levels, but this should be recommended only with careful consideration of energy balance.

Effects on HDL Cholesterol

With weight held constant, decreasing total dietary fat and increasing carbohydrate are associated with reductions in HDL cholesterol levels. Regression analysis predicts a 2.2% reduction in HDL cholesterol for every 5% decrease in total fat in the diet, but individual results vary widely. Often low-fat diets result in greater LDL cholesterol lowering, yielding a significant improvement in the

LDL cholesterol-to-HDL cholesterol ratio. According to some investigators the effects of reducing fat intake on HDL cholesterol level may be relatively small. Compared with an average American diet (37% of energy from fat), a reduced-fat diet was not detrimental for individuals with a low HDL cholesterol level (< 35 mg/dL). In these subjects, the HDL cholesterol level did not decrease on the cholesterol-lowering diet that provided 28% of energy from total fat and decreased only slightly (4%) on the 24% total fat diet. LDL cholesterol decreased substantially (8% and 15% on the 28% and 24% total fat diets, respectively), resulting in an 11% reduction in the LDL cholesterol-to-HDL cholesterol ratio following the 24% total fat diet. In subjects with a higher HDL cholesterol level (> 35 mg/dL), consumption of 28% and 24% total fat diets resulted in a significant decrease in the HDL cholesterol level (8% and 11.5%, respectively), as well as a decrease in the LDL cholesterol level (7.4% and 11.9%, respectively), resulting in an unchanged LDL cholesterol-to-HDL cholesterol ratio.

Similar results have been reported in a heterogeneous group of subjects that varied in age, gender, and ethnicity in the Dietary Effects on Lipoproteins and Thrombogenic Activity study. Both LDL and HDL cholesterol levels were decreased in response to reductions in total and saturated fat, resulting in no significant changes in the total-to-HDL cholesterol ratio. The relationship between HDL cholesterol level and dietary fat must be considered when dietary fat prescriptions are made. For some individuals, a cholesterol-lowering diet that is lower in fat (within the recommended range) may be preferable, whereas for others a diet that is higher in fat (within the recommended range) is more appropriate to beneficially affect the HDL cholesterol level, and, in turn, the ratios of LDL cholesterol-to-HDL cholesterol and total cholesterol-to-LDL cholesterol.

LDL Subclass Patterns

Small, dense LDL (pattern B) increases risk for CHD when contrasted with large, buoyant LDL (pattern A). Approximately one third of individuals who presented with large, buoyant LDL (pattern A) shifted to a pattern B LDL profile (smaller, denser LDL) in response to a diet much lower in total fat and saturated fat. In metabolic ward-type conditions, subjects with pattern A and subjects with pattern B both decreased LDL cholesterol levels when total fat was reduced from 46% to 24% and saturated fat reduced from 183% to 5.4%. The blood lipid lowering was approximately twofold greater for individuals with pattern B compared with pattern A individuals. Reduction in total fat and saturated fat may be especially beneficial for individuals with stable B LDL profile because of LDL lowering potential. A moderate fat level may be more appropriate for individuals with pattern A to avoid a possible shift to pattern B that could occur with dramatic reductions in dietary fat. Weight loss has further been shown to induce a shift from pattern B to pattern A profile. Thus, for some overweight patients with a pattern B profile, a weight-loss diet that is reduced in total fat to achieve an energy deficit may be appropriate if weight loss is achieved and maintained. Alternatively, a moderate diet is more appropriate for weight loss for pattern A individuals to avoid a shift to pattern B, as well as for those subjects with pattern B profile who experienced difficulty with adherence to a weight-loss diet reduced in total fat. Physical activity is encouraged for all cases.

How does the practitioner consider the issue of LDL particle size in the clinical setting? Current methods used in research studies to determine pattern A or B, such as ultracentrifugation, gel electrophoresis, and magnetic resonance imaging, are not routinely run in a clinical laboratory, although development of methods suitable for clinical laboratories is under way. If a patient is very interested, there are specialty laboratories that can determine whether the patient has pattern A or B LDL. In general, pattern B is seen in patients with high triglycerides (> 150 mg/dL) and is uncommon when triglycerides are below 100 mg/dL. Consideration of a patient's subclass of LDL particles could guide the dietitian's final decision on the amount of total dietary fat; however, regardless of particle size, LDL cholesterol is atherogenic. Within the fat allowance, saturated fat should be limited to less than 7% of total energy.

Atherogenic Dyslipidemia

Atherogenic dyslipidemia is characterized by elevated apolipoprotein B and triglycerides, small dense LDL particles, and a low HDL cholesterol level. Often, individuals with atherogenic dyslipidemia are overweight or obese (especially abdominal obesity) and have insulin resistance. ATP III views this atherogenic dyslipidemia as a risk factor because each component (low HDL cholesterol level, small dense LDL particles, and elevated triglyceride-rich lipoprotein and apolipoprtotein B) is individually atherogenic. Beyond LDL cholesterol-lowering strategies, lifestyle changes that promote weight reduction and physical activity favorably modify the components of atherogenic dyslipidemia; such changes are therefore key for treating overweight individuals. An overweight patient with atherogenic dyslipidemia may benefit from a weight-loss diet reduced in total fat to facilitate energy reduction and favorably affect the triglyceride and HDL cholesterol levels. Total fat intake should be individualized to promote adherence and achieve the maximum weight loss possible. Some overweight patients adhere better to a moderate-fat weight-loss diet. Increasing dietary carbohydrate above 60% of energy can reduce HDL cholesterol and increase triglycerides without additional LDL lowering. For normal-weight individuals with atherogenic dyslipidemia, total fat also must be individualized. As previously noted, a diet low in total fat has been shown to benefit persons with a low HDL cholesterol level, as well as persons with a stable pattern B LDL profile. However, because reductions in dietary fat can result in elevated triglycerides, high-fiber foods should be especially encouraged. A moderate-fat diet may be preferable in some patients to potentially raise HDL cholesterol levels, but the emphasis is on lowering triglyceride levels in patients with atherogenic dyslipidemia.

Body Weight

Because dietary fat is calorically dense, decreasing total fat intake can facilitate weight loss. Both the AHA Dietary Guidelines and the National Heart, Lung, and Blood Institute (NHLBI) Evidence Report on the Clinical Guidelines for the Identification, Evaluation, and Treatment of Overweight and Obesity in Adults recommend a total fat intake of no more than 30% as a means of decreasing total energy and facilitating weight loss. The DRI report on macronutrients reviews 10 long-term (> 1 year) weight-loss intervention studies that had a reduced fat intervention. The weight-loss diets provided 12% to 31% energy from fat and resulted in a + 1 to - 6 kg weight change. The National Weight Control Registry (NWCR) reports greater weight loss in individuals who followed self-selected weight-loss programs including a reduction in total fat (eg, 24% of energy). There is also evidence that weight-loss diets moderate in total fat (approximately 35% of energy) achieve long-term weight loss. Obviously, an energy deficit is needed regardless of total fat intake. Collectively, studies conducted to date demonstrate the importance of individualizing total fat recommendations to best achieve weight loss.

NWCR, the largest database of individuals who have been successful in maintaining a substantial weight loss long term (a weight loss of > 13.6 kg [30 lb] that has been maintained for > 1 year), has shown that a modest reduction in total dietary fat is a successful approach to promote weight loss. Of the various dietary strategies used to achieve weight loss, 33.1% of participants limited their percentage of daily energy from fat. Dietary intakes of fat, protein, and carbohydrate as assessed by food-frequency questionnaire were 24%, 19% and 56% of energy, respectively. In addition, individuals maintaining weight loss reported using more behavioral strategies to control their weight, including ongoing adherence to a low-fat diet and exercise regimen and continual monitoring of body weight.

In a study, moderate amount of dietary fat was associated with successful weight los and maintenance of reduced body weight. Weight loss was evaluated in subjects consuming a 20% total fat diet compared with a moderate-fat, Mediterranean-style diet consisting of 35% energy from total fat. The participation rate was only 20% for the low-fat diet group, whereas participation in the moderate-fat diet group was 54% at the completion of the 18-month study. In addition to greater adherence to the diet, the moderate-fat diet group had a greater weight loss at the end of the study (- 4.1 kg), whereas the low-fat group had actually gained weight (+ 2.9 kg). The effects of a formula-based, almond-enriched (39% total fat), reduced-calorie diet compared with a self-selected, reduced-calorie, complex carbohydrate diet (18% total fat) on weight loss has been reported. During this 24-week intervention, subjects following the reduced-calorie, complex carbohydrate diet experienced a plateau at 16 weeks of the weight-loss intervention, whereas those following the almond-enriched diet continued to lose weight for the duration of the trial. These results support other findings documenting difficulties with adherence to a low-fat diet. A moderate-fat diet may offer the most effective approach for weight loss and long-term maintenance of reduced body weight through greater adherence compared with a much lower fat diet (18% to 20% of energy).

A key question for individual patients is "What is the appropriate level of total fat, within the fat recommendation range of 20% to 35%, to promote long-term weight loss and maintenance?" The available evidence suggests that a range of fat-intake levels can be used for successful weight-loss diets. The level of total fat selected is dependent on personal diet-adherence issues and what level facilitates long-term adherence to a calorie-controlled diet. Moderation is the key; dietary fat should not be too low or too high because dietary adherence is challenging with the former, and an adequate energy deficit can be difficult to achieve with the latter.

Glucose and Insulin Levels

It is well established that insulin resistance is a risk factor for the development of hyperglycemia. A high-carbohydrate (i.e., low-fat) diet leads to a greater postprandial glucose and insulin response. The long-term consequences of repeated stimulation of insulin secretion are unknown. Some investigators postulate that it could accelerate beta-cell exhaustion. Moreover, a prolonged elevation in plasma glucose in response to a low-fat, high-carbohydrate diet theoretically could enhance production of glycated products or advanced glycated end products, both of which could be atherogenic. Thus, among individuals who have insulin resistance or type 2 diabetes, it may be prudent for some to follow a higher fat diet within the range recommended by ATP II, as well as the DRI.

Fruits and Vegetables

Fruits and vegetables contain a number of components that may further reduce the development of CHD, including soluble fiber, antioxidant vitamins, folate, and minerals, such as calcium, potassium, and magnesium. However, published data on fruits and vegetables in relation to CHD are limited. Several cohort studies have not confirmed a benefit. The National Health and Nutrition Examination Survey Epidemiologic Follow-up Study did report that CVD mortality for subjects consuming three or more fruits and vegetables per day was 27% lower than for subjects consuming less than one serving per day. Deaths included those due to strokes and ischemic heart disease. Fruit and vegetable intake has also been associated with lower incidence of ischemic strokes.

Although the DASH Study has shown benefits from fruits and vegetables in control of hypertension, trials have not focused on ischemic heart disease. A Finnish 6-week trial provided either a higher polyunsaturated fat diet (using sunflower oil) or a higher monounsaturated fat diet (using high-oleic sunflower and olive oils), with or without the addition of vegetables, berries, and apples. Significant differences in parameters were not observed in serum lipids, homocysteine, and LDL oxidation.

B Vitamins and Homocysteine Levels

Hyperhomocysteinemia (greater than 12 μmol/dL) has been identified as an independent risk factor for CHD. Vitamins involved in homocysteine metabolism (folate, vitamin B-6, and vitamin B-12) are being prescribed by some lipid specialists to normalize homocysteine levels. Polymorphism in the gene for the enzyme methyl tetrahydrofolate reductase (MTHFR), which converts the dimethyl form of tetrahydrofolate to the methyl form (N^5, N^{10} methylene tetrahydrofolate to N^5 methyl tetrahydrofolate), suggest that some individuals may need higher amounts of folate to maintain normal homocysteine levels.

In an effort to reduce neural tube defects, the US government in 1998 mandated that white, refined flour be fortified with 1.4 mg folate for each kg of flour. An additional benefit may be reduction of CHD by lowering serum homocysteine levels. Plasma homocysteine levels were significantly lower in the Framingham population after the initiation of folate fortification of four. Failure to document significantly different homocyseteine levels in a group of Mexican-American women with polymorphisms of MTHFR led to speculation that the now higher intake of folate due to flour fortification may compensate for genetic variations in MTHFR.

Although a number of studies report an association of elevated homocysteine levels with risk for CHD, results from published clinical trials are very limited. Two years of supplementation with 5 mg folic acid and 250 mg vitamin B-6 decreased subclinical atherosclerosis in siblings of patients with CVD. In the Swiss Heart Study, in patients receiving 6 months of supplementation with 1 mg folic acid, 400 μg vitamin B-12, and 10 mg vitamin B-6 after coronary angioplasty, the need for further revascularation was reduced by almost half(20% in those supplemented compared with 38% in the control patients. On the other hand, even though serum homocysteine levels were reduced 18% among CHD patients given 0.5 mg folic acid daily, after 2 years mortality and vascular events were not significantly changed.

How much to supplement? A Danish dose-response study determined 400 μg/day of folate as the minimum dose for adequate homocysteine reduction in 50- to 75-year-old individuals. This is the amount contained in a multivitamin supplement. The Danish population did not have the benefit of folate fortification of flour, as in the United States.

Combining Nutrition Approaches

Having considered the effect of individual dietary factors on risk of CHD, questions arise regarding the potential synergistic benefits from combining these approaches. ATP III estimated the combined impact of its major dietary principles could lower LDL cholesterol levels by 20% to 30%. Studies investigating these overall dietary approaches rather than specific nutrition components are increasingly popular.

In the Lyon Diet Heart Study, provision of a Mediterranean-style diet low in saturated fat, high in monounsaturated and n-3 polyunsaturated fatty acids, and rich in vegetables was associated with a significant reduction in recurrent heart disease. Intervention with a similar diet in India among patients at risk for heart disease found significantly fewer cardiovascular endpoints after 2 years in subjects consuming a diet high in fruits, vegetables, nuts, whole grains, legumes, and n-3 alpha-linolenic acid from mustard seed or soybean oil.

A cross-sectional study of Danish adults classified their diets into three patterns: cosmopolitan pattern (high in fried vegetable, salad, rice, chicken, fish, and wine), a traditional pattern (high in red meat and potatoes, limited in low-fat dairy products and fruit), and a "refined foods" pattern (including french fries, high-sugar beverages, and white bread). The cosmopolitan pattern was associated with higher HDL cholesterol levels and the refined foods with higher total cholesterol levels. A similar comparison of a prudent diet composed of fruits, vegetables, whole grain, and poultry, as contrasted with the Western diet higher in red meats, high-fat dairy products, and refined grains.

Patients with moderate hypercholesterolemia stabilized on a diet with less than 7% saturated fat and less than 200 mg cholesterol per day were then randomized to a control diet, to the experimental portfolio diet, or to use of statin medication. Subjects consuming the dietary portfolio of stanol esters, soluble fiber, soy, and nuts lowered their LDL cholesterol to levels comparable to the levels of subjects receiving the statin medication (28.6% vs 30.9%). In addition, CRP levels were significantly lower in both the dietary portfolio and statin groups than in the control group.

Although nutritional parameters underlie overall dietary approaches to optimize heart health, communication to the public and patients is more meaningful when it focuses on food. As the benefits of including nuts, fish, plant stanol margarines, and many other foods are communicated, attention to substitution rather than addition of foods is important for maintaining energy balance.

PRACTICAL ISSUES IN MNT

On the basis of this research evidence, when the patient's lipid profile and risk factors indicate the need for intervention, MNT is required. Individualized MNT in the clinical setting is currently the most common, but group-based nutrition intervention may also be appropriate and cost-effective in cardiac rehabilitation programs.

In advising patients to adopt these dietary practices, counselors should recognize that some are more easily adopted than others. Using CSFII data and the fat-related questions of the Diet and Health Knowledge Survey, it has been reported that almost half of Americans trim fat from meat, remove skin from chicken, and eat chips infrequently. Although one third of those surveyed used nonfat or low-fat milk, another third never do so. Less-frequent behaviors include use of low-fat cheese and having fruit for dessert.

Individualized MNT Sessions

Provision of MNT through individualized sessions is the most common mode for assisting patients in achieving long-term behavior change. The American Dietetic Association (ADA) offers the Medical Nutrition Therapy Protocol for Hyperlipidemia to standardize the process this protocol is particularly beneficial for reimbursement for MNT. The protocol can be accessed at the National Guideline Clearinghouse Web site (http://guidelines.gov). An analysis of the evidence base for nutrition interventions in hyperlipidemia provides the foundation for the detailed outline of assessment and counseling steps.

The effectiveness of individualized MNT by the dietitian in patients participating in lipid-lowering drug trials has been reported. The investigators reviewed LDL cholesterol levels in patients receiving multiple counseling sessions for stablization on a cholesterol-lowering diet before initiation of medications. LDL cholesterol values were significantly lower after two, three, or four appointments with a dietitian. The trend of declining LDL levels continued beyond the second visit through the third and fourth visits. Approximately half of the patients no longer qualified for lipid-lowering medication according to the earlier ATP II guidelines in effect at the time. This group also reviewed charts of 75 patients with combined hyperlipidemia who participated in an 8-week dietitian intervention program. LDL cholesterol was lowered by 9% and triglycerides by 22%. Cost-benefit data further indicated a saving of $3 in medication cost for every dollar invested in MNT.

In Denmark, a comparison of individuals receiving one brief 10-minute counseling session with individuals receiving two 50-minute sessions found that 1 year later saturated fat intake had decreased significantly (from 11.9% to 9.6% of energy) among subjects receiving the two individualized sessions, but not among those who received only one brief session (10.9% to 10.1%). According to the Cochrane database on evidence-based medicine, the few studies available suggest that nutrition counseling by the dietitian lowers LDL levels more than nutrition intervention by the physician along. The US Preventive Services Task Force recommends intensive behavioral dietary counseling for adults with hyperlipidemia and other risk factors for heart disease. The task force concluded that there is "good evidence that medium- to high-intensity counseling" can produce medium-to-large changes in the average daily intake of saturated fat, fiber, fruit, and vegetables among adult patients at risk for diet-related chronic disease.

Guidelines for MNT Sessions

As outlined by ADA's MNT Evidenced-Based Guide for Hyperlipidemia, an initial MNT session should include assessment, intervention, provision of self-management materials and plans for measuring outcomes. Thorough assessment of clinical data should address risk factors (including smoking history), lipid profile, and medications. Nutrition assessment includes the following:

1. Anthropometric measures, including body mass index (BMI) and waist circumference

2. Biochemical laboratory values, including the lipid profile and serum proteins
3. Change readiness and knowledge for lifestyle changes
4. Dietary assessment, noting
   - Percentage of energy from fat in the diet and types of fat
   - Fiber and viscous fiber intake and sources of fiber
   - Fruit and vegetable intake
   - Use of specific items, such as fish, nuts, soy, and use of stanol- or sterol-fortified products
   - Use of dietary supplements
   - Physical activity levels

The intervention portion of the MNT session should facilitate self-management for identified goals. During this segment, the dietitian does the following:

1. Discuss risk factors
2. Explain role of diet and physical activity in lipid management
3, Provide nutrition prescription based on TLC
4. Explain value of different types of fat
5. Provide information about special food products
6. Discuss self-monitoring techniques, such as food records and pedometers
7. Mutually establish goals, such as those related to serum lipids, BMI, waist circumference, eating behaviors, food intake, and physical activity

Written or Web-based materials should be customized to the client's needs. Patients typically need advice on how to purchase foods and plan and prepare meals, as well as guidance in how to apply principles when eating out, traveling, and celebrating special occasions.

Outcome measures can be derived from assessment data and individualized goals. Follow-up MNT sessions focus on assessment of response to nutrition therapy and the extent to which the patient has been able to adopt recommended lifestyle changes.

Behavioral Issues: Lifestyle Change

Assessment of the patient's stage of change allows for guiding the patient to long-term behavior change. It is helpful to recognize that a patient can be at different stages of change for different heart-healthy behaviors. For instance, a patient may be at the maintenance stage for using nonfat milk, but only at the contemplation stage for eating appropriate portion sizes of meat. Offering patients multiple strategies for dealing with a specific problem food, such as ice cream or bacon, can be helpful. Common strategies include the following:

1. Reducing the portion size
2. Preparing the food more healthfully
3. Reducing the frequency it is eaten
4. Substituting a more healthful food for the problem food

Self-monitoring, such as counting fat grams and recording food intake and physical activity, is essential.

Numerous sample programs, educational materials, and patient resources are available for helping patients achieve a heart-healthy diet. The ADA MNT Evidence-Based Guide for Hyperlipidemia provides materials for use in MNT. Protocols used in clinical trials for reducing heart disease risk and cancer provide excellent ideas. Although developed a number of years ago, the interdisciplinary approach of the Multiple Risk Factor intervention Trial with individual and group sessions continues to provide a model for helping patients to achieve long-term dietary changes with flexible eating patterns. The Polp Prevention Trial, which was designed to reduce recurrence of colon polps, included campaigns to reduce total fat, increase fruit and vegetable intake, and focus on goal achievement. Frequent contact and an action orientation were teamed with novelty, fun, and rewards to enhance achievement of behavior change goals.

Group Classes

Group sessions modeled after clinical trial protocols can be an efficient means of providing nutrition education and counseling to prevent and manage CHD. Target audiences include the general public, individuals with modifiable risk factors for CHD, and cardiac rehabilitation patients (post-myocardial infarction, coronary artery bypass graft, or angioplasty).

Single classes can increase the public's awareness of modifying lifestyle habits for reducing CHD risk and steer them to additional resources, such as Web sites, individual MNT, or a series of group classes. A short series for clients interested in lowering LDL cholesterol levels with dietary strategies could include three to four sessions. When resources permit, a supermarket tour, a cooking demonstration, and tastings can help clients and their families learn to purchase and prepare heart-healthy foods.

CHAPTER 4

CARDIOVASCULAR DISEASE IN SOUTH ASIANS IN USA

It is important to consider health, disease, and cultural factors when developing strategies and tools for the management and prevention of CVD in South Asians in USA. Epidemiologic studies have suggested that individuals of South Asian cultures have a significantly higher prevalence of CHD and several-fold higher rates than other ethnic groups known to have an increased prevalence of CHD. South Asian cultures include people from India, Pakistan, Bangladesh, and Sri Lanka. The term Asian Indian was first designated by the US Census Bureau in 1980 to describe immigrants from the Asian subcontinent. The religions practiced in these cultures have a major impact on eating patterns and lifestyle behaviors. The majority of Indians are Hindus; the majority of Pakistanis and Bangledeshis are Muslims. Other religions practiced in these regions are Christianity, Sikhism, Jainism, Zoroastrianism (Parsis), Buddhism, and Judaism. The majority of the people from Asian-Indian cultures are from India. These groups are among the fastest growing in the United States.

According to data from the 2000 Census, 1.7 million people in the United States identify themselves as Asian Indians. The following statistical profile describes Asian-Indian immigrants in the United States:

1. Five percent of all physicians in the United States obtained their primary medical degree from India.
2. The median family income of Asian Indian households is 25% higher than for all US households.
3. Thirty percent of all hotels and motels in the United States are Indian-owned.
4. Thirty-five percent of Asian Indians live in the northeastern United States, 17.9% in the Midwest, 24% in the south, and 23.1% in the west.
5. Forty-five percent of Asian-Indian women are employed outside the home.
6. Seventy-five percent of Asian Indians were born outside the United States.
7. Eighty percent of Asian-Indian men have college degrees.

Within Asian-Indian cultures, extended family members may live together as a single-family unit. The husband's parents may move in with a family or single siblings and become a part of the household.

Asian Indians in the United States have one of the highest rates of cardiovascular disease. Several studies have also reported a higher incidence of cardiovascular disease among Indian immigrants in England, South Africa and West Indies compared with other ethnic groups. This may be due to high fat diet, high triglyceride, high LDL, high ApoB, low HDL and high homocysteine levels. Indian males develop coronary artery disease to 10 years earlier and have small coronary arteries. Studies have shown that as individuals migrate from a less developed to more developed country, their dietary fat intake increases and cardiovascular disease also increases. This has also been observed among Japanese Americans in California and Hawaii, and among Yemenite jews in Israel and Irish immigrants in Boston. Deaths from cardiovascular disease are very low in Japan. The Japanese consume only 9% of fat from total calories and only 3% from animal fat. When they migrate to America, their diet becomes high in fat, and death from cardiovascular disease increases. Similarly, as Indians migrate to America, their risk of developing cardiovascular disease increases significantly. Enas and his associates conducted a study on the prevalence of Coronary Artery Disease (CAD) and its risk factors in Asian Indians who migrated to the United States. They studied 962 Asian Indian physicians and their families. They completed a questionnaire and screened participants for their lipoprotein and chemistry profile. The data was compared to NHANES, NHIS, and Framingham offspring study. According to this study, lipid profile and other factors of Asian Indians were as follows:

1. High triglycerides
2. Low HDL cholesterol
3. High LDL cholesterol
4. High total cholesterol/HDL ratio
5. High LDL/HDL ratio
6. High APO B
7. High Lipoprotein A LP(a)
8. High APO B/APO A - 1 ratio
9. Dense LDL trait
10. Hyperapobetalipoproteinemia
11. High prevalence of diabetes

According to the Enas et al, high triglyceride, high LP(a), low HDL, and diabetes may have synergetic effects in enhancing the atherogenic effects of LDL. This may make Asian Indians more susceptible to coronary artery disease. Enas et al recommend a LDL of 100 mg/dl for Asian Indians, unless the HDL is high (>60 mg/dl), other risk factors are absent and no abnormalities of lipoprotein or apolipoprotein are found. Prevention should begin early in life. Indians and other ethnic group who migrate to America may not be able to do anything about their genetic make-up, but they can do something about their living conditions. Improved living conditions can be created by abstaining from smoking, reducing stress, exercising regularly and eating a low fat diet.

CVD RISK FACTORS IN SOUTH ASIANS

Lipids and Lipoproteins

High plasma triglycerides and low HDL cholesterol levels have been documented in Asian Indians. Total cholesterol and LDL cholesterol levels in Asian Indians have been shown to be 20 to 40 mg/dL lower than in whites. The frequency of small, dense LDL particles could be an additional coronary risk factor in Asian Indians. Elevation of lipoprotein (a)[Lp(a)], which has been shown to be a strong CVD risk factor, is also present in this population. The presence of these abnormalities is significantly higher in Asian Indians than in European Americans. In addition, South Asians may have a higher risk for CHD from metabolic syndrome (i.e., glucose intolerance, abdominal obesity, hypertension, and dyslipidemia with hyperinsulinemia and insulin resistance).

Diabetes, Impaired Glucose Tolerance, and Hyperinsulinemia

The prevalence of diabetes in Asian Indians is fourfold higher than in whites thereby increasing the risk for CHD. Healthy, normal weight Asian Indians are more likely to have insulin resistance and hyperinsulinemia compared with age- and BMI-matched whites.

BMI and Body Fat

Abdominal obesity characterized by an increased waist-to-hip ratio is prevalent in Asian Indians. Compared with whites, Asian Indians have significantly greater abdominal fat and visceral fat at normal BMIs. Asian Indians have a lower BMI and a higher percentage of body fat than whites. It has been recognized that the relationship between percentage body fat and BMI is ethnic specific. For comparisons of obesity prevalence between ethnic groups, BMI cut points are not appropriate.

Asian Indians may be classified as normal weight but metabolically obese individuals who are prone to diabetes, hypertension, hypertriglyceridemia, and hyperinsulinemia. Other studies have also shown a correlation between insulin resistance and central adiposity in Asian Indians. High abdominal fat in Asian Indians may explain their high risk for CVD and metabolic syndrome. Therefore, lowering the cut points for BMI in these groups may be helpful in the primary prevention of CVD and associated risk factors such as diabetes and hypertension. A routine measurement of waist-to-hip ratio in Asian Indians should be recommended.

Table 1. Pattern of Dyslipidemia among Asian Indians Relative to American Whites

Lipid	Relative Serum Concentration
Total Cholesterol	Similar
LDL	Similar
Small, Dense LDL	Higher
Trigylcerides	Higher
HDL	Lower
Lp(a)	HIgher

Several cholesterol abnormalities help explain the prevalence of CHD in the Asian Indian population. The common pattern of dyslipidemia seen in Asia Indians when compared with the lipid profiles of white Americans is listed in Table 1. Asian Indians tend to have higher triglycerides, lower high-density lipoprotein (HDL), higher lipoprotein(a)[Lp(A)], and small, dense low-density lipoprotein (LDL) particles, also known as LDL Pattern B.

National Cholesterol Education Program Adult Treatment Panel III (NCEP ATP III) guidelines establish the acceptable "normal" level of triglycerides as < 150 mg/dL. In the United States, however, 43% of Asian Indian males and 24% of Asian Indian females have levels that exceed 150 mg/dL.

An HDL of 60 mg/dL is considered optimal in both whites and Asian Indians. HDL is deemed low when it drops below 40 mg/dL. However, most experts regard a level of < 50 mg/dL to be low in women. A study of Asian Indians living in the United States found that 54% of men had HDL below 40 mg/dL, and 68% of women had levels below 50 mg/dL.

The cardioprotective effects of HDL are mostly confined to large HDL particles (HDL2). Small HDL cholesterol (HDL3) is not only associated with less protection against atherosclerosis, but also with increased progression of atherosclerosis. At a given level of cholesterol, the concentrations of large HDL cholesterol (HDL2) were lower and concentrations of small HDL cholesterol (HDL3) were significantly higher in Asian Indian men than in Caucasian men. The overall HDL particle size was smaller in Asian Indians than whites. These abnormalities may represent dysfunctional HDL that is not ascertained by the conventional lipid profile.

Lp(a) also is a major risk factor in Asian Indians, which could explain the high incidence of early myocardial infarctions in this population. Elevated Lp(a) is a genetic risk factor that has been shown to at least double the risk for a heart attack. Although Lp(a) > 30 mg/dL is generally considered the threshold at which risk of premature CHD increases rapidly, levels below 20 mg/dL are considered optimum, particularly in Asian Indians. Studies of Asian Indians in North America found that 23-50% of sampled populations have levels > 30 mg/dL. This level corresponds with > 10 mg/dL of Lp(a) cholesterol as measured by the VAP Test. Furthermore, LDL Pattern B is a risk factor in any population, but it is particularly prevalent in Asian Indians. Small, dense LDL particles can be more easily oxidized and penetrate the artery wall much more efficiently than larger LDL particles.

Finally, the constellation of risk factors that make up the metabolic syndrome contributes to the increasing incidence of CHD in Indians. In particular, the atherogenic lipid triad of the metabolic syndrome – low HDL, high triglycerides, and small, dense LDL (Pattern B)– is the hallmark of insulin resistance. Since rates of diabetes are very high in Asian Indians, the disease further contributes to heart disease risk in this population.

Asian Indian Women & CHD

Asian Indian women have a higher rate of CHD than do women of other ethnic groups, despite similar conventional risk factors and lipid profiles, and the rate is growing. According to a recent study of coronary heart disease mortality for six ethnic groups, from 1990 to 2000 death rates for heart disease among women in California declined with the exception of Asian Indian women, who experienced a 5% increase.

A study conducted by Bhalodkar, et al., found that LDL cholesterol concentrations were similar in Asian Indian women compared with Caucasian women from the Framingham Offspring Study, but Asian Indian women had smaller HDL particle sizes despite having similar HDL-C concentrations. Small HDL particle size may partly explain the excess burden of CHD in Asian Indian women.

The Role of the VAP Test

The VAP Test provides a tool to identify lipid risk factors in the Asian Indian population that the routine cholesterol test misses. In a single test, the VAP Test provides the information found in a routine lipid panel, plus measurements of all known cholesterol subclasses that play important roles in the development of CHD, including Lp(a), LDL pattern density, and the metabolic syndrome. The VAP Test improves the ability to identify heart disease risk to more than 90%, compared with just 40% with the routine cholesterol test. The VAP Test also provides a more accurate, directly measured LDL, as recommended in the NCEP ATP III guidelines.

The VAP Test & Treatment Options

In addition to lifestyle modifications, such as increasing physical activity and eating a diet low in fat and cholesterol, appropriate drug therapy should be considered for all lipid abnormalities that do not respond to lifestyle adjustments. The VAP Test's breakdown of lipid subfractions is vital in determining appropriate treatment options for the Asian Indian population. The availability of more sophisticated cholesterol treatments points to broader use of the VAP Test because results will help physicians more specifically match a drug or combination of drugs with a patient's cholesterol profile.

While statins are the therapeutic cornerstone for reducing major coronary events, they primarily affect LDL. Triglycerides are only modestly decreased, and HDL is only slightly elevated. In addition, statins have little or no effect on Lp(a). As a result, additional drug therapies such as nicotinic acid should be considered for treatment of Asian Indians and others with these important, emerging CHD risk factors. Niacin is a safe and effective medication that lowers Lp(a) and triglycerides and increases HDL, particularly the large cardioprotective HDL particle. In addition, a patient's response to therapy should be checked with a follow-up VAP Cholesterol Test 6-12 weeks after starting drug therapy in order to make any needed adjustments or additions.

The epidemic of CHD in Asian Indians is starting to be recognized in the medical community, and the need to minimize its toll is apparent and vital. Physicians and community members must work to increase awareness, particularly among the younger generation, that heart disease is preventable. Women should be particularly aware of the problem, and preventive measures such as exercise, diet and pharmacologic solutions should be implemented. The VAP Test can detect risk factors that studies have shown to be most prevalent, including elevated Lp(a), a small HDL, and LDL Pattern B. A combination of preventive measures and customized treatment options can help reverse the devastating effects of heart disease on this population.

Homocysteinemia and C-Reactive Protein

Plasma homocysteine is an independent risk factor for Asian Indians and may contribute to their increase CHD risk. Compared with Europeans, Asian Indians' fasting homocysteine concentrations were 6% higher. In the same study, Asian Indians were found to have lower vitamin B-12 and folate levels. Reduced intake of vitamin B-12 has been reported in Asian Indians. Vitamin B-12 levels have been found to be significantly lower in Indian men and women in the United States; especially in Indian men compared with non-Indian men. In addition, prolonged cooking of vegetables in South Asian households destroys a significant amount of dietary folate.

Elevated CRP levels occur in a number of Asian-Indian adults and adolescents. Both high CRP levels and generalized and abdominal obesity may contribute to metabolic syndrome and atherosclerosis in Asian-Indian adults.

HEALTH BELIEFS AND FOOD SELECTION

Holy scriptures generally guide the food selections of people in Asian-Indian cultures. For example, the Vedic scriptures, followed by Hindus, describe connections between types of foods and longevity, fitness, and mood. Milk and milk products (excluding cheese made with rennet), wheat, rice, legumes, certain vegetables, and ghee (clarified butter, a source of saturated fat) are associated with health, longevity, and serenity. Meats, eggs, and foods of extreme tastes, such as bitter, sour, and salty, are associated with passion and aggressive behavior.

The Ayurveda system of Indian medicine is based on the belief that foods can provide a homeostatic harmony or cause imbalance. Ayurvedic remedies for gastric illnesses include such foods as papaya and eggplant to improve digestion. Moderation is recommended to prevent obesity.

Vegetarianism is practiced by large sections of the Asian-Indian population and is based on being nonviolent to all beings. Most Hindus are lacto-vegetarians. Beef consumption is forbidden in Hinduism. Jaines, in addition to being strict lacto-vegetarians, do not eat root vegetables such as onions, garlic, beets, carrots, and potatoes. They do not eat between sunset and sunrise. Many vegetarian foods, including desserts, are often prepared with butter, ghee, hydrogenated fats (vanaspati), coconut oil, and palm kernel oil. Sikhism permits meat consumption, and Parsis consume fish, eggs, shrimp, chicken, and goat. Eggs are symbols of fertility, and fish is considered to be an auspicious food. Muslims follow koranic laws that permit the consumption of meats of certain animals sacrificed in a humane way known as halal. If the meat is not obtained according to the Islamic law, it is forbidden, or haram. Haram foods also include pork, alcohol, meat from clawed animals, and fish without scales. Crustaceans such as shrimp and lobster are considered undesirable, or makruh.

Fasting is an important religious practice among Asian Indians. Hindus follow partial fasting rituals throughout the year, and Muslims observe a month of complete fasting during which neither foods nor fluids are consumed from dawn until sunset. This fasting period is known as Ramadan, the ninth month of the lunar calendar. Pregnant and lactating mothers and sick people are exempt. They can postpone the days for fasting, or, if they are unable to do so, they can feed the poor in accordance with the law.

Spices and herbs are an essential component of Asian-Indian cuisines. Some spices are used in the treatment of ailments. Ginger is recommended for nausea and motion sickness; fenugreek is believed to prevent hyperglycemia in type 2 diabetes.

Other countries near India, such a Sri Lanks, Nepal, and Bhutan, have common dietary patterns and practices in addition to their distinct foods. In India alone, food practices vary depending on the region. The regional practices are described in the American Dietetic Association publication Indian and Pakistani Food Practices, Customs, and Holidays and on the America Association of Physicians of Indian Origins Web site. The common features of Asian-Indian diets include the following:

1. Rice and wheat are staples and can be prepared with large amounts of saturated fats such as butter and ghee or with the use of hydrogenated fats containing trans fatty acids. Rice dishes include pilaf, biriyani, and wheat preparations such as puris, paratas, and naan. These breads are either deep fried or topped with ghee and butter after cooking.
2. A large variety of legumes, including chickpeas, black-eyed peas, and lentils, are used in the preparation of curries such as dal and sambar, in combination with vegetables, with meat, and in papadums. Legumes fried in hydrogenated fat and oils, commercially available, are also consumed as snacks, usually with midafternoon tea.
3. Meat, poultry, fish, and eggs are prepared as curries or kebabs and in combination with grains (biriyani), legumes, or vegetables. Coconut milk, butter, ghee, and vegetable fats can be used to stir fry and improve texture and flavor. The spices and herbs used in the Asian-Indian cui-

sine can be a variety of combinations, depending on the region and type of recipe. This means all curries are not created equal.

4. Vegetables are prepared with onions, garlic, spices, oil, butter, cream, or yogurt. Potatoes or legumes are usually cooked with vegetables (for example, spinach with potatoes; zucchini with lentils.
5. Fruits are eaten as desserts, snacks, as an appetizer with spices and salt (chat), or in combination with yogurt as a drink (mango lassi).
6. Dairy products such as yogurt cheese (panir), yogurt, and milk are used as ingredients in the preparation of rice dishes (biriyani), with vegetables (palak-panir), in desserts, or as an accompaniment to the meal.

Eating Patterns and Nutrient Intake

In a study of 187 Indian men of a particular community living in the United States, fat represented 36% of the subjects' energy intake, their saturated fat intake was greater than that of Indian men not living in the United States, and their intake of fiber (14 g/day) was below the recommended dietary allowance. In a study of 153 Asian-Indian male physicians, the average energy intake included 56% from carbohydrate, 32% from fat, and 8% from saturated fat. High total fat was significantly associated with increased triglyceride levels. In the same study, an uneven distribution of food during the day (skipping breakfast and eating large dinners) was associated with high plasma triglyceride and low HDL cholesterol levels. South Indians have low plasma levels of alpha-linolenic acid, eicosapentaenoic acid, and docosahexaenoic acid. However, the high coronary risk in Asian Indians is not fully explained by unfavorable characteristics of their eating patterns.

Physical Activity

Studies have reported that South Asians are less likely to incorporate exercise in their daily living habits, and physical inactivity has been associated with abdominal obesity.

Studies of South Asians' attitudes toward lifestyle changes in the prevention and treatment of CVD are limited. A focus group study on South Asian women in England suggested that barriers to lifestyle changes included lack of knowledge about ways to cook ethnic foods healthfully and the unavailability of women-only exercise facilities. Focus group participants perceived stress as an important risk factor for CHD. They had problems accessing health and leisure services because of language and cultural barriers.

In general, South Asians eat their own foods for dinner and prefer more convenient foods such as cereals, sandwiches, and pizza for breakfast and lunch.

In the larger cities, high-fat home-style meals are purchased from Indian and Pakistani restaurants.

ATP III GUIDELINES TO ASIAN INDIANS

The ATP III guidelines state that absolute risk for CHD may vary in different racial and ethnic groups, but relative risk from risk factors is similar for all population groups. ATP III guidelines apply to African Americans, Hispanics, Native Americans, Asian and Pacific Islanders, and South Asians. Beyond lowering LDL cholesterol levels, metabolic syndrome is a secondary target of therapy in the ATP III guidelines. As Asian Indians become acculturated to American diets and lifestyles, several factors can contribute to metabolic syndrome. These include overweight and obesity, physical inactivity, and high-carbohydrate diets (> 60% of energy intake) in some persons. Underlying genetic factors also contribute.

To reduce CVD risk, reducing obesity and increasing physical activity are valuable steps. In addition, one should treat associated lipid and nonlipid risk factors: hypertension, prothrombotic state, and atherogenic dyslipidemia.

DIETARY RECOMMENDATIONS

A low-fat, high-carbohydrate diet may not benefit Asian Indians because it may accentuate metabolic abnormalities (high plasma triglycerides, low HDL cholesterol, and the presence of insulin resistance). Medical nutrition therapy should focus on the following:

1. Intensifying weight management (reducing abdominal fat). Make daily exercise a priority; learn ways to work out at home; use a pedometer for feedback; and eat high-fiber cereal breakfast with nonfat milk and fruit.
2. Decreasing carbohydrate intake, particularly refined carbohydrates. Use whole-grain flour (millet or whole wheat) to make breads such as chaptis and naan, brown rice to prepare pilaf and other rice dishes, and oat and whole-wheat breakfast cereals to prepare savory snacks.
3. Increasing intake of n-3 fatty acids. Mix flax seed powder in curries (eg. sambar), dal (lentil soup), vegetable dishes, or chapatis; eat fenugreek leaves (methi) as a vegetable; consume fatty fish such as salmon (if religion permits); and use canola oil and walnuts in food preparation.
4. Decreasing intake of saturated fat, trans fatty acids, and cholesterol. Use canola oil or extra-light olive oil in place of butter, ghee, vanaspati (hydrogenated fat), and margarine; substitute almond paste or nonfat yogurt for cream and butter in buttery makhani curries; use low-fat milk

(1% fat) to prepare yogurt cheese panir; and substitute egg whites for egg yolks in omelets and desserts.

5. Optimizing protein intake. Eat fresh or frozen soybeans as savory snacks (chole, chat, sundal) and in combination with vegetables such as spinach and zucchini; cool tofu with tomatoes, spinach, onions, or with nonfat yogurt as raitha.
6. Increasing intake of fruits and vegetables. Choose fruits as snacks, instead of fried legumes such as bhel; substitute green leafy vegetables for potatoes with legumes.
7. Decreasing intake of salt. Use herbs such as cilantro and mint; cook with spices such as cumin, black pepper, cardamom, and cinnamon that enhance food flavors.
8. Optimizing intake of calcium and vitamin D. Consume nonfat milk, nonfat yogurt, and nonfat milk powder in combination with fruit as shakes and dessert.

Table 2. Food habits and adaptation in USA by South Asians

Group	Comments	Common Foods	Adaptation in the United States
ASIA INDIAN			
PROTEIN FOODS Milk/milk products	In general, milk is considered a beverage for children. Fermented dairy products are popular.	Fresh cow's, and buffalo's milk; evaporated milk; fermented milk products (yogurt, lassi); fresh curds very popular, milk-based desserts, such as kheer, khir, kulfi, barfi; butter, especially clarified (usli ghee)	More cheese consumed; ice cream popular
Meats/poultry/fish/ eggs/legumes	Sophisticated vegetarian cuisine; legumes primary protein source. Eighteen varieties of beans, peas, and lentils commonly used. Collectively, legumes called pulses. Chickpeas and lentils known as dals. Legumes are typically prepared whole or pureed, or used as flour to prepare baked, steamed, for fried breads and pastries.	**Meats**: beef, goat, mutton, pork **Poultry**: chicken, duck **Fish and seafood**: Bombay duck, clams, crab, carp, herring, mackerel, mullet, pomfret, sardines, shrimp, turtle **Eggs:** chicken **Legumes:** beans (kidney mung, etc), chickpeas, lentils (many varieties and colors), peas (black-eyed, green)	Consumption of legumes decreases; meat intake increases. Meat may be added to traditional vegetarian dishes. Fast foods are popular.
CEREALS/ GRAINS	Over 1,000 varieties of rice are cultivated. Wheat used mostly in the North; rice in the South. Most breads (roti) are unleavened.	Rice (steamed, boiled, fried puffed), wheat, buckwheat, millet	Use of American-style breads in place of roti

FRUITS/ VEGETABLES	Over 100 types of fruit and 200 types of vegetables are commonly used. Fruits and vegetables may be used in fresh or preserved pickles called, rayta (northern), pachadi (southern), or chutney.	Fruit: apples, avocados, bananas (several types), coconut, dates, figs, grapes, guava, jackfruit, limes, litchis, loquats, mangoes, melon, nngus (fruit of the palmyra), oranges, papaya, peaches, pears, persimmons (chicos), pineapple, pomegranate, pomelos, raisins, starfruit, strawberries, sugar cane, tangerines, watermelonVegetables: agathi flowers, artichokes, amaranth, banana rhizome, bamboo shoots, beets (leaves and root), bitter melon, brussels sprouts, cabbage, carrots, cauliflower, corn, collard greens (haak), cucumbers, eggplant, lettuce, lotus root, manioc (tapioca), mushrooms, mustard greens, okra, onions, parsnips, plantain flower, potatoes, radishes (four types, leaves and roots), rhubarb, sago palm, spinach, squash, sweet potatoes (leaves and roots), tomatoes, turnips, yams, water chestnuts, water lilies	Decreased variety of fruits and vegetables available; decreased vegetable intake. More fruit juice is consumed. Salad is well accepted. Use of canned and fozen produce increases.

ADDITIONAL FOODS Seasonings	Aromatic (northern) and hot (southern) combinations of fresh or dried spices and herbs accentuate or complement food flavors.	Ajwain (carob seeds), amchoor (dried ground mango), asafetida (a powdered resin), bay leaf, cardamom) (two types), chilis, fresh coriander, cinnamon, cloves, coconut, coriander seeds, cumin, dill, fennel, fenugreek, garlic, kewra (essence of screwpine flowers), limes, lemon, mace, mint, mustard, nutmeg, pepper (black and red), poppy seeds, rose water, saffron, tamarind (a type of bean), turmeric	Spice use depends on availability
Nuts/Seeds	Nut and seeds of all types are popular; used to thicken korma sauces.	Almonds, betel nuts and leaves, cashews, peanuts, pistachios, sunflower seeds, walnuts	Paan tray may be limited to betel nuts and spices.
Oils		Coconut oil, ghee, mustard oil, peanut oil, sesame seed oil	Purchased ghee often made from vegetable oil instead of butter
Sweeteners		Sugar cane, jaggery (unrefined palm sugar), molasses	Candy and sweets enjoyed, but not overconsumed.

Table 3.Healthier Versions of Traditional Asian-Indian Cuisine

TRADITIONAL FOOD	HEALTHIER ALTERNATIVES
Meat, poultry, fish, and eggs fried in ghee, butter, coconut oil, palm kernel oil, or hydrogenated fats and oils	Bake, roast, broil, grill, or oven-fry. Remove skin from chicken before eating. Fry with canola, olive, or corn oil. Limit oil to 1/4 cup.
Legumes and vegetables prepared with oil, butter, cream, or yogurt to enhance flavor.	Use almond paste or nonfat yogurt in place of cream and butter. Season with onion, garlic, spices, or low-sodium chicken broth to enhance flavor.
Rice (white) dishes or wheat (refined) preparation deep-fried or prepared with large amounts of ghee, butter, and hydrogenated fats (vanaspati) containing trans fatty acids.	Use brown rice and whole-grain wheat. Boil or bake instead of frying. Fry with canola, olive, or corn oil or with trans fat-free margarine instead of solid or hydrogenated fat.
Whole milk, cheese, cream, or yogurt used to prepare rice dishes, vegetables, desserts, and shakes; yogurt cheese (panir) prepared with whole milk.	Use low-fat or nonfat milk, milk powder, cheese, cream yogurt, buttermilk, or soymilk.
Omelets and desserts prepared with egg yolks.	Substitute egg whites for egg yolk.
Snacks such as fried legumes (bhel)	Snack on fruits, rice cakes, and puddings made with low-fat milk instead. Use oat and whole wheat cereal to prepare savory snacks.
Salt used to enhance flavor	Use herbs (eg, cilantro, mint) or spices (eg, cumin, black pepper, cardamom, cinnamon).

CHAPTER 5

RECIPE FOR A HEALTHY HEART

1. Maintain an appropriate body weight

   Obesity is associated with number of health problems; as discussed in an earlier section of this book. A strong correlation exists between body weight and blood pressure. Obesity makes it easier for genetic abnormalities to manifest themselves.

2. Reduce total fat intake in the diet to less than 30% of total calories. Cook with little or no fat. Avoid frying foods. Instead stir-fry, broil, microwave, broil, roast or steam your food. Use more vegetables and fruits.

3. Reduce saturated fats to less than 10% of total calories. Reduction of saturated fat in the diet also reduces total cholesterol. Tropical oils like coconut, palm, kernel, ghee (clarified butter) are very high in saturated fat. They are frequently used in commercially prepared crackers, snacks and Indians sweets. It is important to read labels before buying your favorite snacks. Hydrogenated oils (margarine etc.) should be limited in the diet. The hydrogenation process saturates fats and changes their chemical structure and this tends to raise total blood cholesterol. Substitute liquid oils for solid shortening in cooking.

4. Polyunsaturated fats should comprise up to ten percent of total calories. Rich sources of these oils include safflower, sesame, sunflower, corn and soybean. These oils can help lower blood cholesterol levels.

5. Monounsaturated fats should comprise up to 15 percent of total calories. Rich sources of these fats are olive, canola, peanut and avocado. Studies have shown that monounsaturated oils help reduce cholesterol levels.

6. Cholesterol intake should be less than 300 milligrams per day. A normal adult manufactures about 1,000 milligrams a day. The remaining cholesterol comes from animal food sources. The body needs small amounts of cholesterol for cell membranes and some hormones. Saturated fats and dietary cholesterol raise blood cholesterol levels. The American Heart Association has developed two plans for people who have high cholesterol levels. The Step One Diet is for healthy people whose cholesterol

levels are slightly high. Step two diet further reduces saturated fat to 7 percent of calories and dietary cholesterol to less than 200 mg a day.

7. Reduce simple carbohydrates (sugars) to 10-15% of total calories. These include rich desserts and cookies.

8. Increase complex carbohydrates to 50-60% of total calories. Some water-soluble dietary fibers such as oat bran, pectin (found in apples, oranges, and grapefruit), and guar gum (found in beans, peas, and lentils) have a cholesterol lowering effect. Water insoluble fibers, such as wheat bran do not have this property. High fiber diet can also be helpful in losing weight. In our Bariatric Clinic at Howard University, we have been using high fiber diets in the treatment of obesity. Patients on these diets loose significant weight. Fiber slows the absorption of food and this gives a feeling of fullness. The best way to increase fiber in the diet is to eat fruits, especially apples, oranges and grapefruit. Oat bran, beans, peas, and lentils are also effective. The diet of most South Asians includes lentils. They can improve their diet by not using saturated fats in lentils and eating more fruits and vegetables. Another way they can increase fiber content is by adding oat bran flour to their chappatis (bread). It is recommended that the diet should include 20-30 grams of fiber per day. It is important to increase water intake with high fiber intake.

9. The American Heart Association recommends that healthy adults not consume more than 2400 mg of sodium per day. Some people with high blood pressure need to reduce their salt intake further. One teaspoon of salt contains 2,000 mg of sodium. Canned, precooked foods, pickles, salted nuts, prepared soups and desserts are very rich in sodium.

10. Alcohol — A number of studies have shown that alcohol raises HDL cholesterol (good cholesterol) levels. Some studies have shown that this increase is mainly in HDL_3 rather than HDL_2 (the protective component of HDL cholesterol). Therefore, it is recommended that if you don't drink, don't start because the benefits are negligible. If you do drink, limit your intake to 2 drinks a day (1 ounce ethanol) of wine, beer or liquor.

11. Do not smoke. Cigarettes greatly increases an individual's chances of developing heart disease. Smoking decreases HDL cholesterol (good cholesterol) and is associated with the development of atherosclerosis.

12. Exercise. Regular physical activity reduces the risk of cardiovascular disease. It increases HDL levels, lowers triglyceride levels, improves

glucose tolerance, reduces high blood pressure, controls weight, and lessens depression. The amount and intensity of exercise varies with different individuals. An individualized exercise program should be developed in consultation with your physician. In healthy individuals, an exercise program of moderate intensity (e.g. brisk walking) thirty to forty-five minutes a day five days a week is recommended.

13. Stress. A number of studies have shown that stress increases LDL cholesterol (bad cholesterol). It is recommended that you keep your stress level low by minimizing frustrating and angry situations and making time for pleasurable activities. Meditation can be very helpful in reducing stress as mentioned earlier in the book.

CHAPTER 6

NUTRITION LABELS

The nutrition Labeling and Education Act "passed by the requires food products to carry labels called Nutrition Facts. The label provides the following information:

1. Serving size
2. Servings per container
3. Calories per serving
4. Total fat per serving
5. Saturated fat per serving
6. Cholesterol content
7. Sodium content
8. Total carbohydrates
9. Dietary fiber
10. Sugars
11. Protein
12. Vitamin A
13. Vitamin C
14. Calcium
15. Iron
16. Percent daily

Percent daily values are based on a 2000 calorie diet.
Following are some words frequently used in labels.

1. Calorie free — less than 5 calories per serving
2. Light (lite) — one third less calories or half the fat of the high-calorie food or high fat food, or half the sodium of high sodium food.
3. Fat free — less than 0.5 grams of fat per serving
4. Low fat — 3 grams of fat per serving
5. Reduced or low fat — 25% less fat
6. Lean — less than 10 grams of fat, 4 grams of saturated fat and 95 mg of cholesterol per serving

7. Cholesterol free — less than 2 grams of cholesterol and less than 2 grams of saturated fat per serving
8. Low Cholesterol — less than 20 mg of cholesterol and 2 grams of saturated fat per serving
9. Sugar free — less than 0.5 grams of sugar per serving
10. High fiber — 5 grams or more of fiber per serving
11. Sodium free — less than 5 mg of sodium per serving and no sodium chloride in the product
12. Very low sodium — 35 mg or less of sodium per serving
13. Low sodium — 140 mg or less of sodium per serving
14. Reduced or less sodium — 25% less sodium than the original amount in product

In addition to reading labels, it is also important to read ingredients. Ingredients in the greatest amount are listed first, and ingredients in the least amount are listed last. Reading the ingredients will help you avoid getting too much fat or sodium. Sources of fat and cholesterol in packaged foods are as follows:

1. Animal fat
2. Bacon fat
3. Butter
4. chicken fat
5. Lard
6. Lamb fat
7. Pork fat
8. Turkey fat
9. Hardened fat
10. Beef fat
11. Ham fat
12. Egg and egg yolk solids

Sources of saturated fat are: cocoa butter, coconut, coconut oil, hydrogenated vegetable oil and palm oil. Some of the acceptable ingredients are: sunflower oil, corn oil, canola oil, soybean oil, sesame oil, olive oil, safflower oil, skim milk, nonfat dried milk solids, and diglycerides. The other ingredient you should look for is sodium. If you are supposed to avoid sodium, you should carefully read the label's listing of ingredients.

If one does not choose food carefully, the South Asian Diet can be dangerously high in total fat, saturated fat, cholesterol and sodium. For example, Ghee (clarified butter) is frequently used in Indian and Pakistani food. Ghee is very high in fat and cholesterol. South Indian food is high in coconut which is a very rich source of saturated fats. Sweets are also extremely rich in cholesterol and saturated fats because they are prepared from whole milk and ghee. Indian and Pakistani pickles are very high in sodium. Chinese food is also high in sodium if monosodium glutamate (MSG) is used in cooking. Some South Asian canned and packaged now have labels similar to American labels. Read them carefully.

CHAPTER 7

EATING OUT

People are eating out more frequently. According to a 1993 survey, Americans are spending about 43 percent of their food dollars on foods purchased away from home. People eat out either from necessity or for pleasure. Eating out frequently means that an individual's diet will be high in fat, cholesterol and sodium. Even though many restaurants have started offering low fat dishes, one must be very careful still in making choices. Some of the concerns about eating out frequently are as follows:

1. Fats. High fat ingredients include cheese, butter or oil and the fat is all the more harmful when dishes are deep fried or sauteed.
2. Portions. Portion sizes are very large. One is tempted to overeat.
3. Sodium content is high. This may be due to the use of excessive salt, or the use of ingredients that are high in sodium.
4. Fiber-rich foods are not used. Instead, meat and poultry are featured while fiber-rich foods are used as side dishes.
5. Beverage intake tends to be high, especially beer, wine, hard liquor or carbonated beverages.

Strategies For Eating Out

1. Avoid foods that are high in fat and saturated fat. Avoid breaded, fried, buttered, creamed, escalloped and au gratin dishes. Good choices are au jus, baked, barbecued, broiled, poached, steamed or roasted dishes.
2. Order sauces and salad dressings on the side.
3. Divide the meat portion into two servings. Eat one and take the other home.
4. Ask for skim or low fat milk for coffee or tea.
5. Be careful when using extra salt. Some people with high blood pressure are sensitive to salt. Be aware that ketchup, mustard, pickles and tartar sauce are high in sodium.
6. Avoid croissant and biscuit sandwiches. They are very high in fat.
7. For dessert, select sherbet or fruit.

Asian American have also changed their eating habits by eating out frequently or ordering taxi out foods. Some Asian American favorite eating places follow:

Chinese

Most Asian Americans are fond of Szechuan or Hunan type Chinese cooking that features chillies, garlic and hot red peppers. Some similarities appear with Indian and Pakistan cooking. Whether the food is high in fat, sodium and calories will depend on what you order. Foods high in fat are: Duck, cashews or peanuts, egg, and bits of pork used in cooking. And, of course, dishes that are lightly fried, breaded or deep fried contains more fat.

Foods recommended in Chinese restaurants are: streamed or stir fried vegetables, meats cooked in hot and spicy tomato sauce or served on a sizzling platter. Chinese food is high in sodium unless you specifically request that you do not want MSG (Monosodium Glutamate) used in your dish. Specific dishes recommended in Chinese restaurants are as follows:

Appetizers
Steamed dumplings
Roast Pork strips
Beef or chicken satay

Soups
Hot and sour
Wonton
Sizzling rice with chicken or shrimp

Chicken
Hunan spice chicken
Chicken with vegetables
Chicken chop suey
Chicken stir fried with Chinese cabbage/vegetables

Meats
Beef and broccoli
Twice cooked pork
(Pork with cabbage, green peppers and other vegetables
Roast pork with vegetables

Seafood
Shrimp with tomato sauce
Shrimp with broccoli

Vegetables
Vegetarian delight
Spicy green beans
Broccoli & black Mushroom

Rice
Steamed White

Noodles
Roast Pork low mein
Chicken low mein
Vegetable low mein

Desserts
Lychee nuts
Ripe apple crunch

Indian Pakistani

Indian and Pakistani restaurants are growing in numbers in the United States. Their cuisine includes a variety of spices, vegetables and legumes. Rice and bread are important parts of the meal. This type of cuisine is high in fiber and low in animal protein. However, the problem is that lots of fat, especially ghee (clarified butter) is used in the cooking. Some dishes contain coconut which as we have already stressed, is a rich source of heart-harmful saturated fat. Many breads like pooris are deep fried, and popular appetizers, for example, pokara and samosa are also deep fried. Dishes especially recommended from Indian and Pakistani restaurants follow:

Appetizer
Papad
Chicken Tikka

Soup
Mulligatamy
(Lentils, vegetables)
Vegetables
Dahl Rasam
(Pepper soup
with lentils)

Chicken
Chicken tandoori
(Marinated in spices & roasted in a clay oven)
Chicken saag
Chicken with skimach
Chicken masala
(Roasted chicken cooked in spices)

Meat
Lamb bhuna
(roasted lamb with spices & onions)
Lamb saag
(Lamb cooked with spinach)
Kheema matar
(minced lamb and peas)

Seafood
Shrimp curry
Fish vindalloo
(Fish with potatoes
& hot spices)

Vegetables
Aloo chole
(Chick peas with potatoes)
Razma (kidney beans)
Vegetable curry
Bhartha
(Roasted eggplant cooked in spices)
Dhal (lentils with spices)

Rice
Plain boiled
basmati rice

Breads
Chappati
Nan (without ghee)

Dessert
Fresh fruit

Fast Food

Fast food places offer low-priced foods and quick service. Many fast food restaurants have started offering salad bars, baked potatoes, beans and sugar free soft drinks. Be cautious in choosing foods from fast food restaurants! Generally, fast foods are high in fat, saturated fat and sodium. The nutrient content of these foods is given in the table at the back of this book. Recommended foods from the fast food restaurants are:

1. Plain hamburger with tomato, lettuce (no mayonnaise). Avoid the cheese, bacon and ham
2. Grilled chicken sandwich
3. Chef salad with low fat dressing
4. Baked potato with chilli and light cheese
5. Low fat frozen yogurt
6. Thin "n" crispy pizza
7. Grilled vegetarian pizza

Foods to Avoid in Fast Food Restaurants:

1. Fried chicken
2. Croissant sandwiches
3. Biscuit sandwiches
4. Sauces
5. Bacon
6. Cheese sauce
7. Sour cream
8. Salad dressing (regular)
9. Breaded and fried foods
10. Fried desserts
11. Fried foods
12. Double and triple decker burgers

Mexican Food

The fat content of Mexican foods is very high. Popular foods include nachos with guacamole, cheese and sour cream, tacos, cheese enchiladas and refried beans. Healthy choices are soft chicken tacos, chicken or beef fajitas. Some Mexican restaurants have stared offering "Border Lights". These foods include chicken tacos, taco salad, bean and beef burritos, all excellent choices because they contain half the fat of the regular menu.

Recommended Mexican foods follow:

1. Tostado with hot salsa
2. Black bean soup
3. Chili con carne
4. Gazpacho
5. Mexican salad
6. Taco salad
7. Fajitas
8. Enchiladas
9. Burritos
10. Tostadas
11. Chili verde
12. Mole Pollo
13. Anozcon Pollo
14. Mexican Rice
15. Black beans
16. Tortillas (flouror corn)
17. Flan

CHAPTER 8

THE GOOD HEALTH DIET

Dairy Products

Eat Less	**Substitute**
For 1 C Whole Milk	1 C Skim Milk
For 1 C Plain Yoghurt	1 C Nonfat Yoghurt
For American, Cheddar, and Blue Cheese	Low-fat Cheese, Skim Ricotta or Mozzarella

Breads

	Use instead
For Croissants, butter rolls	English muffins, bread sticks
For doughnuts, muffins	Whole grain breads
For Parantha, puri (Indian bread)	Chappati (without ghee or butter)

Meats

Eat Less	**Substitute**
Beef, Lamb, Pork	Fish, Turkey, Chicken

Fats

Eat Less	**Substitute**
Butter and Spread	Oil (sparingly)
Ghee	
Butter, margarine or ghee for frying or sauteing	Vegetable Oil

Desserts

Eat Less	**Substitute**
For 1 C Ice Cream	1 C nonfat frozen yogurt, ice milk, sorbet, or ice pops
For 1 slice pecan pie	1 slice apple pie
For Chocolate cake with icing	Angel food cake
For 2 Chocolate chip cookies	2 Vanilla wafers
Indian sweets (mithai) made with ghee, whole milk and sugar	Home-made "mithai" with lowfat milk

Other Substitutions

1 ounce potato chips	1 ounce pretzels (low fat)
1 C buttered popcorn	1 C air-popped popcorn
1 ounce chocolate	3 marshmallows
1 ounce peanuts or cashew nuts	2 C air-popped popcorn
1 slice pepperoni pizza	1 slice vegetarian pizza
1/4 C sour cream	1/4 C non-fat plain yogurt
1 C cream of tomato soup	1 C vegetarians split pea soup
1 tablespoon mayonnaise	1 tablespoon mustard
1 tablespoon heavy cream	1 tablespoon non-dairy cream

Helpful Shopping

- Always shop from a list. Resist *"impulse"* buying.

- Never shop when you are hungry. That's when will power is at its lowest.

- Allow extra time to read labels. Look for food low in fat and sodium and high in fiber.

Helpful Cooking

Meat

- Trim visible fat off before and after cooking.
- Remove poultry skin.
- Roast, bake or broil the meat.
- Meat can be basted with vegetable oil instead of butter.
- Do not use butter or heavy cream sauces. Substitute low fat yogurt.

Vegetables

- Steam or stir-fry in vegetable oil.
- Do not use butter or ghee in frying vegetables.

Desserts

- Begin a life-long love affair with fresh fruits. They are **ALWAYS BETTER** than rich desserts.
- Make your own desserts at home. In this way you can control the ingredients and make smart substitutions — for example, oil instead of butter or ghee and nonfat yogurt instead of for heavy cream.

Breads (Indian/Pakistani)

- When making parantha, always use vegetable oil.
- Fry poori in vegetable oil.
- It is always best to substitute nan or chappatti; (without butter or ghee) for parantha or poori.
- Always use whole wheat floor. You can add oat bran to increase fiber content.

Small Steps When You Eat Out

Be aware that restaurant food is usually high in saturated fat.

- Ask for salad dressing on the side so that you can control the amount.
- Choose nan without butter or ghee instead of parantha and pari.
- Choose boiled basmati rice over palao.
- Choose tandori chicken or shishkabab.
- If you choose a curried dish, use the curry sparingly.
- Ask for sauteed vegetables instead of vegetable curry dishes in cream sauce.

South Asian Cooking

- Use vegetable oil instead of ghee or butter.
- Use margarine sparingly as a spread instead of butter.
- Use low-fat yogurt instead of whole yogurt.
- Prepare your meats in the oven or grill.
- Use low-fat yogurt instead of heavy cream.
- Use nuts sparingly in the cooking.
- Use oil for "tadka" in the dal.
- Use coconut sparingly in the cooking.
- Use salt sparingly.
- Make sweets at home so you can control ingredients like fat and sugar.

Ways to Increase Fiber in Your Diet

- Use whole wheat bread instead of white bread.
- Use brown rice instead of white rice.
- Eat fruits and vegetables with skin.
- Increase consumption of whole beans, kidney beans, chick peas, pinto beans and navy beans.
- Mix oat bran flour with regular flour to make chappatis.

HEALTHY HEART RECIPES

BREAKFAST FOODS
Cereals with Skim Milk

Name of Breakfast Cereal	Amount of Cereal	Amount of Milk	Calories	Fat gm	Cholesterol gm	Fiber gm
1. Oatbran	3/4 cup	1 cup	166	3.4	4	5
2. Shredded Wheat	2 biscuits	1 cup	256	10.4	4	6
3. Wheat bran	1/4 cup	1 cup	116	1.4	4	7
Snackwell (fat free)	**bar**		**Calories**	**Fat gm**	**Cholesterol mg**	**Fiber gm**
1 bar			120	0	0	1
1 cup skim milk			86	.4	4	-

CRACKED WHEAT PORRIDGE

Ingredients

2 T	cracked wheat (dallia)
1/4 t	fat (optional)
1 ½ C	water
1 C	skim milk
1 t	sugar

Method

1. Roast wheat dallia in a pan, using little oil if necessary, until lightly brown.
2. Add water and bring to boil. Cook on slow fire, stirring occasionally, until well done and thick in consistency.
3. Serve hot in a bowl or soup plate with skim milk and sugar.

Yield:	1 serving
Serving Size:	1 cup
Calories per serving:	110
Total Fat:	1 g
Cholesterol:	4 mg
Fiber:	0.2 gm

Yogurt & Fruit

Ingredients

1 C	nonfat yoghurt
½	Banana
1/4 C	strawberries
2 T	Oat bran (instant)

Method

Place all ingredients in a blender and puree.

Yield:	1 serving
Serving Size:	1 bowl
Calories per serving:	229
Total Fat:	2.2 g
Cholesterol:	4 mg
Fiber:	4.5 g

SUJI UPMA

Ingredients

1T oil	3T suji (semolina)
1 pinch asfatida (hing)	water (double the volume of suji)
1/4t mustard seeds	½ t salt
1/4t urad (washed)	1/6t red chili powder (optional)
1 whole red chilli	½ finely chopped green chilli
1 sprig curry leaves	1/2 t lemon juice
1/8" ginger	1 small onion

Method

1. Heat oil in a wok or frying pan, fry hing, splutter mustard seeds, fry urad dal to a golden brown color, fry whole red chilli and curry leaves.
2. Add semolina and roast to pink color on a very slow fire.
3. While suji is roasting, boil double the volume of water as that of semolina, add salt and red chilli powder.
4. Add roasted suji to the boiling water slowly and steadily, stirring constantly to avoid lump formation (the fire being kept at moderate flame while mixing is being done). Cook till the mass is dry. Serve hot garnished with chopped green chillies, coriander leaves and a sprinkle of lemon juice.

Yield:	2 servings
Serving Size:	1 bowl
Calories per serving:	151
Total Fat:	5.5 g
Cholesterol:	0.0
Fiber:	-

SCRAMBLED EGGS

Ingredients

½ medium onion	1 chopped green chilli
2 T oil	1/4 C egg beater
2 T peas	Salt and pepper to taste
½ medium size tomato	1 t ginger grated
1/4 small green chilli	

Method

1. Fry chopped onions, ginger, chilli in oil in a frying pan. Add tomatoes and green peas.
2. Pour egg beater and mix slowly until the mixture looks like scrambled eggs.

Yield:	1 servings
Serving Size:	1 bowl
Calories per serving:	50
Total Fat:	10 g
Cholesterol:	0
Fiber:	12 g

SOUPS

MIXED STOCK

Ingredients

½ lb bones and chicken trimmings (without skin)
3 C water 1 small onion
1 small carrot

Method

1. Break bones and chop chicken into small pieces. Add water and other ingredients and cook them for 1 ½ hour.
2. Pour through a colander to remove the solids. Do not rub.
3. Cool the stock and remove the hard fat from top.

Yield:	2 cups
Serving Size:	1 cup
Calories per serving:	35
Total Fat:	0.5 g
Cholesterol:	0.2 mg
Fiber:	0.1 g

Vegetable stock - substitute various vegetables

MINESTRONE SOUP

Ingredients

½ small onion	½ clove garlic
½ small carrot	1 bay leaf
1 leaf cabbage	1T spaghetti, macaroni or noodle
½ medium tomato	1/8 t pepper
1 t oil	1 t salt (seasoning)
	Garnish coriander leaves

Method

1. Chop onion, shred cabbage and dice carrot fine.
2. Heat oil in a saucepan, add onion and carrot, saute.
3. Add stock, bring to boil. Add macaroni, skinned and chopped tomato and bay leaf.
4. Simmer gently for 20 minutes. Add the cabbage and seasoning.
5. Cook until the vegetables are soft.
6. Garnish with coriander leaves.

Yield:	1 serving
Serving Size:	1 bowl
Calories per serving:	80
Total Fat:	1.5 g
Cholesterol:	0.3 mg
Fiber:	0.6 g

CHICKEN SWEET CORN SOUP

Ingredients

½ lb chicken	1T water
2 C stock	salt and pepper - to taste
small corn on the cob	1 egg white or egg substitute
1 ½ t cornflour	

Method

1. Boil the chicken in stock for 20 minutes. Put the stock aside and shred the chicken.
2. Grate the corn on the cob, add stock and cook for 20 minutes.
3. Add shredded chicken mixture (keep some chicken shreds for garnishing) and bring to boil again.
4. Make paste of cornflour with water. Add it to the soup and cook for 3 minutes, stirring constantly.
5. Add salt and pepper and when the mixture is simmering, add the lightly beaten egg white or egg substitute. Stir with a fork in one direction to create "threads" of egg white.
6. Pour soup into deep serving bowl and serve hot, garnished with chicken shreds.

Yield:	1 serving
Serving Size:	1 bowl
Calories per serving:	300
Total Fat:	3 g
Cholesterol:	75mg
Fiber:	1.3 g

SPINACH SOUP

Ingredients

1 t oil	1/4 t salt
1/4 small onion	1/8 t pepper powder
½ clove garlic	a pinch nutmeg powder
3 ½ oz. chopped spinach	1 t flour

1 ½ cup vegetable or chicken stock

Method

1. Gently sauté finely chopped onion and crushed garlic in oil for 5 minutes.
2. Add the chopped spinach and cook gently until tender.
3. Stir in flour, then whisk in the stock. Bring to boil and season with salt, pepper and nutmeg powder.
4. Cover and simmer for 30 minutes.
5. Sieve or liquidize and strain. Return to pan, bring back to boil and add the seasoning.

Yield:	1 serving
Serving Size:	1 bowl
Calories per serving:	100
Total Fat:	5 g
Cholesterol:	0
Fiber:	0.7 g

VEGETABLE DAL SOUP

Ingredients

2	T olive oil	2	onions, chopped
1	green bell pepper, diced	1	carrot, pared and diced
1	clove garlic, minced	2	small zucchini, grated
3	C stock (meat or vegs for broth)	2	C water
2	C cooked dal (lentil)	1	C canned puree tomatoes
1	bay leaf	½	t oregano
½	t salt	½	t curry powder
1	C cooked brown rice	1	T lemon juice
1	T fresh coriander for garnishing		

Method

1. Heat oil. Add onion, pepper, carrot, garlic and saute. Add zucchini and cook for an additional 7 minutes.
2. Add stock or (chicken, broth), water, dal, tomatoes, and bay leaf. Bring to a boil over medium heat. Reduce heat to medium and simmer for 15 minutes.
3. Add salt, pepper and simmer 10 minutes longer. Add rice. Remove from heat and add lemon juice. Garnish with coriander leaves.

Yield:	5-6 servings
Serving Size:	1 bowl
Calories per serving:	190
Total Fat:	3 g
Cholesterol:	0
Fiber:	6.5 g

GARAM MASALLA
(Fresh Ground Spices)

Ingredients

2 t freshly ground cardamon
4 t cinnamon sticks, broken into pieces
8 t whole cloves
4 t peppercorns
4 t black cumin seeds
1/4 t nutmeg powder
2 t freshly ground seeds from large black cardamon

Methods

1. Grind the cinnamon, cloves, peppercorns, and black cumin seeds and seeds from large cardamon in a blender.
2. Mix together the freshly ground spices with the nutmeg powder, and ground cardamon. Shake the container to mix the spices thoroughly. Yields about 2 tablespoons.

(This spice is also available in Indian stores. If you do not have time, you can purchase it ready made.)

PANIR
(Home Made Cheese)

Ingredients

2 quarts (2%) milk
2 T lemon juice
½ C low fat (2%) yogurt

Method

1. Bring milk to a boil. Reduce heat to low and stir in lemon juice and yogurt. Stir until milk curdles. Remove from heat immediately.
2. Strain through cheese cloth.
3. Spread mixture to form circle or square, and put heavy weight on it.
4. Leave for 2 to 3 hours.
5. Remove from cheesecloth.
6. Cut into small pieces.

(Some Indian stores carry ready made cheese.)

THESE TWO RECIPES, PANIR AND GARAM MASALLA ARE GIVEN AS THEY ARE FREQUENTLY USED IN THE FOLLOWING RECIPES.

DAHI ALOO
(Potatoes & Yogurt)

Ingredients

1 small potato	1/4 t turmeric powder
2 t oil	1/4 t garam masala
½ Medium onion	1/4 c low fat yogurt
1/8" ginger	salt to taste
½ Green chilli	1/8 t chilli powder (optional)
1 Small tomato	chopped coriander leaves for garnishing
½ t coriander powder	½ c water

Method

1. Boil potatoes. Drain, peel and cut in small pieces. Saute` in oil until slightly brown. Drain and set aside.
2. Chop the onion finely; mince the ginger and chilli very finely and chop the tomato.
3. Heat the remaining oil and fry the onion until soft but not brown.
4. Add ginger, coriander powder, turmeric and garam masala and fry for five minutes.
5. Add chillies, tomato and yogurt. Stir until the gravy begins to thicken. Then add water, salt and chilli powder.
6. Simmer until gravy is thick.
7. Add the boiled potatoes and cook for a minute or two.
8. Garnish with chopped coriander leaves.

Yield:	1 serving
Serving Size:	1 bowl
Calories per serving:	267
Total Fat:	12 g
Cholesterol:	4 mg
Fiber:	1.1 g

STUFFED KARELAS
(Bittergoud)

Ingredients

3	medium karelas	a pinch red chilli powder
½ t	salt	a pinch turmeric powder
for Masala		1/4 t mango powder (amchur)
2 t	oil	1½ T oil (to shallow fat fry)
1	clove garlic (crushed)	1/8 t salt

Method

1. Scrape, wash and make a length-wise slit in the karela. Put salt over the surface and inside slit and leave for 2-3 hours.
2. Wash karelas well and squeeze out the bitter juice.
3. Fry the masala to a golden brown color and add mango powder; cook till dry.
4. Fill the slit karela with this mixture; tie a thread around it.
5. Shallow fat fry to a golden brown color on all sides; drain off excess fat.
6. Untie the thread and serve hot.

Yield:	1 serving
Serving Size:	3 Karelas
Calories per serving:	366
Total Fat:	33 g
Cholesterol:	0
Fiber:	1.7 g

PEAS AND CABBAGE

Ingredients

2 t ginger	1/8 t red chilli powder (optional)
1/4 cabbage, medium size	1/4 t turmeric powder
½ c peas	1 green chilli
1T oil	A few coriander leaves
½ t salt	1/8 t garam masala

Method

1. Chop ginger, shred cabbage.
2. Fry ginger until golden brown.
3. Add salt, red chilli powder, turmeric and green chilli. Fry lightly and add cabbage and peas. Cook lightly, stirring occasionally for 2 - 3 minutes and then cover.
4. Sprinkle chopped coriander leaves and garam masala.

Yield:	1 serving
Serving Size:	1 bowl
Calories per serving:	212
Total Fat:	5 g
Cholesterol:	0 g
Fiber:	3.3 g

CABBAGE ROLLS
(Dry or Curried)

Ingredients

2 large or 4 small cabbage leaves
1 green chilli, chopped
1 t oil
2 T ground turkey or ground chicken
1 onion
2 T crumbled low fat cheese (paneer)
1 clove garlic
1/4 t lemon juice
2 t ginger (minced)
A pinch of salt

Method

1. Wash the cabbage, separate the leaves carefully and remove the hard stem, if needed. Steam until the leaves are half cooked.
2. Heat oil and saute lightly the finely chopped onion, garlic, ginger and green chilli.
3. Add mince meat or paneer, salt, red chilli powder and cook until tender, adding 2 T water if required. Allow to cool and divide into two parts.
4. Spread the cabbage leaves on a wooden board. If they are small in size, place two of them with one edge overlapping.
5. Put one part of the minced meat/paneer mixture on one edge of each leaf (or on overlapping pair of leaves), roll and turn the sides gently in.
6. Sprinkle a little lime juice seasoned with a pinch of salt and pepper over the rolls.
7. Roll in dry flour and shallow fry or bake in a moderately hot oven (325°F) after spraying with oil.
8. For curry - saute ginger chilli, add the rolls and 1 t water and cook for 2 minutes. Add tomato puree and cook for 2 minutes.

Yield:	1 servings	
Serving Size:	2 rolls	
Calories per serving:	meat, 341;	paneer, 350
Total Fat(g):	23;	28
Cholesterol (mg):	12;	5
Fiber:	1.5	1.5

EGGPLANT (BAINGAN) BHARTHA

Ingredients

1 small eggplant	½ t salt
1 small onion	1/4 t red chilli powder
1 small tomato	1/4 t garam masala
1 small green chilli	a sprig green coriander (chopped)
1 t oil	½ t ginger, minced

Method

1. Broil the eggplant.
2. Peel, wash and mash well.
3. Chop onion, tomato and green chilli.
4. Fry the onions lightly and add tomatoes, green chilli and seasoning.
5. Add the mashed eggplant and cook until dry and glossy.
6. Serve hot, garnished with coriander leaves.

Yield:	1 serving
Serving Size:	1 bowl
Calories per serving:	187
Total Fat:	5 g
Cholesterol:	0
Fiber:	3 g

STUFFED TOMATO

Ingredients

2 firm tomato	2T low fat cheese
1 small potato	½ t salt
1 carrot	1/4 t red chilli powder
½ cup peas	1/4 t garam masala
½ onions	2 t Oil
1 t fat	A sprig chopped coriander leaves

Method

1. Cut off a thin slice of tomato from top and keep it aside. Scoop out the pulp and keep it aside. Drain off tomatoes and sprinkle a little salt into the cavities.
2. Boil, peel and cut potato and carrot into small pieces.
3. Chop onions fine.
4. Heat oil, fry onions lightly. Add tomato pulp, cooked vegetables, paneer and seasoning. Cook till well mixed and a little dry. Add coriander leaves and remove from fire.
5. Fill the tomato sheets with this mixture. Replace the tomato caps.
6. Bake in a very moderate oven (325°F) for about 5-7 minutes. (Brush pan with a little oil before baking).

Yield:	1 serving
Serving Size:	2 tomatoes
Calories per serving:	288
Total Fat:	5.5 g
Cholesterol:	2.3 mg
Fiber:	2.5 g

OKRA (Bhindi)

Ingredients

½ cup okra	1/4 t salt
1 small onion	1/8 t red chilli powder
1 teaspoon oil	1/4 t turmeric powder
	1/8 t coriander powder

Method

1. Wash and dry or wipe bhindis with a wet cloth.
2. Cut them into half-inch slice and slice the onion into long thin pieces.
3. Heat oil in a teflon pan, gently put in the bhindis. Cook open stirring occasionally.
4. When half done and less sticky, add onions and seasoning. Stir.
5. Cook covered on a slow fire until done and crisp.

Yield:	1 serving
Serving Size:	1 bowl
Calories per serving:	105
Total Fat:	4.6 g
Cholesterol:	0
Fiber:	1.6 g

CURRIED CARROTS

Ingredients

2 medium size carrots, cut into small pieces
1/8 t cumin seeds
1 t oil
pinch salt
1 small green chilli, cut into small pieces
pinch pepper
½ t grated ginger

Method

Heat oil, add cumin seeds, green chilli, ginger. Saute 5 minutes.
Add carrots. Stir let mixture stay on low heat about 10-15 minutes.

Yield:	1 serving
Serving Size:	1 bowl
Calories per serving:	80
Total Fat:	4.6 g
Cholesterol:	0
Fiber:	4.5 g

LENTILS - PULSES (Dals)

Dal (lentil) With Squash (ghia)

Ingredients

4 ½	Channa Dal	1 t	cumin powder
4 C	water	1 t	coriander powder
3 C	chopped ghia or green squash peeled, chopped)	3/4 t	turmeric powder
		1/4 t	*garam masalla*, a spice mixture
1/8	teaspoon *asafetida (heeng)*	1 T	vegetable oil
1 t	minced garlic	4	Dried red chilies
1/4 t	chili powder	½ t	*amchoor*, powdered mango
1 T	coriander		

Method

1. Remove stones from the dal. Wash the dal thoroughly and soak in water for 1 hour in a heavy bottomed pot.
2. Add chopped ghia, asafetida, minced garlic, chili powder, powdered mango, coriander powder, and turmeric powder. Stir well and bring to a boil. Reduce heat to moderate, partially cover, and cook for 1 hour. (Can be cooked in the crock pot).
3. Add garam masalla, stir well, reduce heat to low, and simmer, tightly covered, another 30 minutes.
4. In a skillet, heat the oil and saute the chilies, frying until the chilies become very dark.
5. Transfer contents of the skillet to the pot, stir once, and simmer, uncovered, 4 to 5 minutes. Garnish with coriander.

Yield:	6 servings
Serving Size:	1 bowl
Calories per serving:	175
Total Fat:	2.3 g
Cholesterol:	0
Fiber:	1 g

Sambar

Ingredients

2 T	tamarind pulp	1 ½ C	diced eggplant
2 ½ C	hot Water	1 ½ C	chopped okra
1-1/4 C	arhardal (lentil)	1	tomato
6 C	water	1 C	drumsticks
1 t	tumeric powder	3	curry leaves or bay leaves
1/4 t	asfetida	3 T	oil
½ t	fengureek seeds	2	green chillies, chopped
½ T	corriander seeds	2	whole red chilli
2 ½ t	cumin seeds		
salt to taste			

Method

1. Soak tamarind in ½ C of hot water for 30 minutes and extract the pulp.
2. Clean and wash dal. Add tumeric powder. Add 5 cups of water and soak for half an hour. Then cook over moderate heat until dal is soft. Cover mixture partially for 45 minutes or you can prepare cook.
3. Add the eggplant, okra, drumsticks to the cooked daal. Cook 15 minutes. Add the tamarind juice. Stir and cook for another 15 minutes.
4. Soak tomato in 2 C hot water, peel and chop. Add to the daal.
5. Roast corriander seeds, fengureek seeds, cumin seeds, and grind. Add to daal.
6. In the skillet, heat the oil. Put asfetida and mustard seeds. Fry until they spultis, add curry leaves, green chillies, red chillies, fry 2 minutes and then add to daal mixture.

Yield:	6 servings
Serving Size:	1 bowl
Calories per serving:	164
Total Fat:	7.5 g
Cholesterol:	0
Fiber:	2 g

Rasam

Ingredients

1-1/4 C	arhardal (lentil)	1/4 t	asfatida
1/4 C	boiling hot water	2 ½ t	cumin seeds
2 T	tamarind pulp	1 ½ T	corriander seeds
5 C	water	4	corn pepper
2	whole red chillies	1	tomato
1 t	mustard seeds	1 t	tumeric powder
2 T	oil	1 T	corriander leaves
salt to taste		3	curry leaves

Method

1. Soak tamarind in hot boiling water - extract pulp.
2. Cook daal in 5 C water.
3. Roast red chilli (1), corriander seeds, pepper corns, cumin seeds and grind.
4. Mash the cooked daal. Add ground masala, tamarind, water, salt and peeled, chopped tomato. Cook for fifteen minutes.
5. Heat oil, cook mustard seeds until they sputter. Add red chilli, curry leaves. Add to mixture. Garnish with corriander.

Yield:	6 servings
Serving Size:	1 bowl
Calories per serving:	74
Total Fat:	2.8 g
Cholesterol:	0
Fiber:	1 g

CURRIED RED KIDNEY BEANS (Rajma)

Ingredients

1-3/4 C	red kidney beans	3/4 t	grated ginger
2 t	Chilli powder	1 t	coriander powder
1 t	minced ginger	1 t	cumin powder
½ t	minced garlic	1-½ C	chopped tomatoes (without skin)
3/4 t	turmeric powder	3/4 t	garam masalla
2 T	vegetable oil	2 T	chopped coriander leaves
2 C	finely sliced onions		salt to taste
1 t	grated garlic	2 T	chopped coriander leaves

Method

1. Wash and soak the rajmah over night. Add ½ teaspoon of baking soda.
2. Wash rajmah thoroughly.
3. Put rajmah, salt, red chilli, ginger and garlic in 4 cups of water.
4. Pressure cook the rajmah for 45 minutes or cook a crock pot. Then let it cool and drain the rajmah and reserve the stock separately.
5. Grind onion to fine paste and fry it in heated oil until brown.
6. Add turmeric powder and coriander powder. Fry for 2 minutes.
7. Put in skinned tomato pieces.
8. Add the drained rajmah and fry for another five minutes. Add rajmah masala. Add reserved stock and cook for 20 minutes until gravy thickens.
9. Garnish with chopped coriander leaves.

Yield:	6-8 servings
Serving Size:	1 bowl
Calories per serving:	376
Total Fat:	5 g
Cholesterol:	3 g
Fiber:	1.1 gm

You can add Beano drops to the curry to avoid possible discomfort due to gas.

ALU CHAAT
(Spice Potato)

Ingredients

1 lb	potatoes	1/8 t	black pepper
2 T	tamarina	½ t	cumin powder
1 C	hot water	1/8 t	chili powder
1/8 t	asafetida (*heeng*)	2 t	lemon juice
½ t	vegetable oil	½ t	sugar and
3	small green chilies	1 t	molasses
1/8 t	ginger powder	chopped coriander leaves	

Method

1. Boil potatoes, peel and cut into small pieces.
2. In a wok, heat oil and add asafetida. Next, add the tamarind juice, sugar, molasses, ginger powder, black pepper, cumin powder, and chili powder. Cook over moderate heat about 8 minutes. Lower heat and simmer until the juice thickens (about 10 minutes). Remove from heat.
3. Add lemon juice to the tamarind juice. In a bowl, combine the potatoes and tamarind sauce and mix thoroughly. Transfer to a serving bowl and garnish with coriander leaves and chilies.

Yield:	3 servings
Serving Size:	1 bowl
Calories per serving:	250
Total Fat:	1 g
Cholesterol:	0
Fiber:	1.1 g

VEGETABLE KOFTAS

Basic Recipe for Gravy
Ingredients

1/4 t	Dry coriander seeds	1/8 t	Cumin seeds
1	Medium ground onion	1/8 t	Chilli powder
1/8 t	Salt	1/8 t	Turmeric powder
1	Small tomato (pureed)	½ c	Water
1T	Low fat buttermilk*	3/4 t	Chopped coriander leaves
2	Cloves garlic	1/8 t	Garam masala
1 t	Ginger	2 t	Oil

Method (Preparation of gravy)

1. Grind garlic, ginger, coriander seeds and cumin seeds to a fine paste.
2. Heat and fry ground onion to a golden brown color. Remove pan from the heat and add chilli, salt and turmeric powder.
3. Return to heat and continue frying with addition of 1-2 t water two to three times.
4. Add ground garlic and fry for another five minutes.
5. Add tomato puree and continue frying until fat separates.
6. Add ½ C water and simmer for 15 minutes in a closed pan over low heat.
7. Add koftas, simmer for five minutes. Add buttermilk.
8. Serve garnished with chopped coriander, a sprinkle of garam masala.

Buttermilk should be low fat. Nonfat will curdle.

GHIA KOFTA

(Green Long Squash)

Ingredients (for Koftas)

1/4 lb	Ghia	½	Green chilli
1 t	ginger	1	Clove garlic
1/8 t	garam masala	1/4 t	salt
2 t	chick peas flavor (besan)		

Method

1. Scrape, wash and grate ghia. Boil in 1/3 C water (minimum amount) until just tender (about 10 minutes).
2. Squeeze. Reserve the water for gravy.
3. Add chopped green chilli, ginger, garlic and season. Add besan and shape into 3-4 balls.
4. Preheat oven to 350°. Put oil into the baking pan. Bake until brown on both sides.
5. Add koftas to gravy. Simmer for five minutes.
6. Add low fat buttermilk and garam masala.
7. Garnish with coriander leaves.

Yield:	1 serving
Serving Size:	4 koftas
Calories per serving:	200
Total Fat:	15 g
Cholesterol:	0
Fiber:	1.7 g

GREEN BANANA KOFTA

Ingredients (for Kofta Mixture)

1 big green banana
1/4 t salt
1 t finely sliced ginger
2 cloves chopped garlic
½ finely cut green chilli
½ brown cardamon (crushed)
1/8 t garam masala
½ t finely chopped coriander leaves
3 t chick peas flour (Besan)
For gravy - same as basic recipe

½ C water (enough to cover bananas)
2 t oil

Chopped nuts (optional) as below

2 almonds
pistachio nuts, chopped
2 vaisino
1 T oil for sauteing
2 t low fat milk

Method

1. Boil the bananas with the skin intact in the boiling salted water for about 10 minutes or till tender. Allow to cool.
2. Peel, mash the banana thoroughly.
3. Heat 2 t oil and lightly fry the onion, garlic and ginger.
4. Add the banana pulp, salt, green chilli, cardamon seeds, garam masala and finely chopped coriander leaves. Stir for a few seconds and cool.
5. Mix milk and besan and knead until mixture is a pliable dough.
6. Divide the mixture into four balls with the help of a little oil in your hands.
7. Make a depression in the center, put a little nut mixture, if used, into this depression. Close and re-form into balls.
8. Saute under medium heat until golden brown. Remove from fat and drain.
9. Prepare gravy as in Basic Recipe.
10. Put koftas in a serving dish and pour hot gravy over it.
11. Sprinkle with coriander leaves

Yield:	1 serving
Serving Size:	4 balls
Calories per serving:	340
Total Fat:	15 g
Cholesterol:	0
Fiber:	2 g

LOTUS ROOT KOFTAS

(Kamal Kakri Kofta)

Ingredients

For Kofta Mixture

Canned lotus root
2 cloves chopped garlic
1 small chopped green chilli
1/4 t salt
1 t chopped ginger
1/8 t garam masala
1 T besan chick pea flour
1 T besan
oil for saute
For gravy - The same as for Kela Kofta

Method

1. Mince lotus root.
2. Thoroughly mix the remaining ingredients listed under kofta mixture with the lotus root to make a pliable dough.
3. Divide the mixture into 3-4 equal parts with the help of a little oil. Shape into balls.
4. Saute koftas in non-stick frying pan.
5. Put kofta in a serving dish and pour hot gravy over it.

Yield:	1 serving
Serving Size:	4 koftas
Calories per serving:	400
Total Fat:	20 g
Cholesterol:	0
Fiber:	26 g

KEEMA MATAR

Ingredients

1 T	oil	½ t	salt
1	clove	1/4 t	turmeric
½"	Stick cinnamon	1 t	ginger
1	Brown cardamon	2	cloves garlic
1	Small onion	2	peeled, chopped tomatoes
1/8 t	chilli powder	½ C	peas
½ lb	ground turkey	2 T	water
1	bay leaf	½	(finely cut) green chilli
		A sprig	coriander leaves

Method

1. Roast clove, cinnamon and cardamon.
2. Remove immediately from heat and crush.
3. Heat oil and fry the onions until golden brown.
4. Remove from the heat, add red chilli powder and a teaspoon of hot water.
5. Place on slow heat and cook until water is absorbed.
6. Add the turkey, bay leaves, crushed whole spices, salt and turmeric. Cover, stirring occasionally until the juices in the mince dry up.
7. Grind ginger and garlic, add to the mince and cook for about 5 minutes.
8. Add blanched, peeled and chopped tomatoes.
9. Cover and cook until the tomatoes are mixed up with the mince, and gravy thickens. Add peas and fry for a few minutes. Add water.
10. Return to heat and simmer until done.

Yield:	1 serving
Serving Size:	1 bowl
Calories per serving:	300
Total Fat:	10 g
Cholesterol:	75 mg
Fiber:	3 g

CHICKEN- DO-PIAZA

Ingredients

1 small onion	**For masala**
1 t oil	1 t oil
1/4 t salt	1 small onion
1/3 t chilli powder	3 cloves garlic
2 t coriander powder	1 bay leaf
2 T low fat yoghurt	1 green cardamon
150 g chicken	2 t water
	1/4 t garam masala
	A sprig of coriander leaves

Method

1. Heat oil in a wok and add finely chopped onion, salt, chilli powder, coriander powder, yogurt and chicken.
2. Cook on low heat until onions become soft and meat is tender (or pressure cook for 10 minutes and dry the liquid). Lightly fry the meat.
3. For masala, heat oil and add chopped onion, garlic, and bay leaf. Fry to golden brown color.
4. Add the above meat-onion mixture, crushed green cardamon and water. Cook on gentle heat for 5 minutes.
5. Serve hot, garnished with garam masala and chopped coriander leaves.

Yield:	1 serving
Serving Size:	1 bowl
Calories per serving:	250
Total Fat:	11 g
Cholesterol:	75 mg
Fiber:	.1 g

SEEKH KABABS (Turkey)

Ingredients

1/4 lb	ground turkey
1/4 t	salt
1 t	Lime juice
1/4 t	poppy seeds
1	Almond
½ t	cumin seeds
1/4 t	low fat yoghurt
1/8 t	Red chilli powder
1/8 t	garam masala
1	clove
1 t	coriander seeks
3	Pepper corns
1 t	grated ginger
a pinch	nutmeg
1/4 t	water
a few	coriander leaves

Method

1. Add salt and lime juice to meat and set aside for one hour to allow the mince to become tender.
2. Roast poppy seeds, almond, cumin seeds, cloves, coriander seeds and pepper corns on a griddle.
3. Grind these with ginger, nutmeg and add low fat yoghurt.
4. Mix with minced meat, add red chilli powder and garam masala.
5. Add water and knead hard for a few minutes as this makes the paste sticky and suitable for holding on the skewers.
6. Chop coriander leaves finely and add to the paste.
7. Divide into 4 long sections and flatten them.
8. Pass skewer through the center of each part, and using a moistened hand, fold the meat on to it.
9. Rotate the skewer slowly and press the meat gently with fingers moistened with a little water, until it completely circles the skewer.
10. Leave for 10 minutes and roast on a charcoal fire or in an oven.
11. Turn slowly when one side is done. Do not turn too frequently. Grill until the kababs they are evenly browned on all sides.

Yield:	1 serving
Serving Size:	4 kababs
Calories per serving:	200
Total Fat:	10 g
Cholesterol:	75 mg
Fiber:	0.2 g

BUTTERMILK CHICKEN

Ingredients

1 t	Oil	1/4 t	Salt
1	Small onion, finely chopped	1 ½ t	Sugar
1 t	ginger, grated	2 T	Low fat butter milk
2	cloves garlic	1/4 t	Garam masala
½ t	Red chilli powder	2 pieces	tandari chicken
2	Peeled tomatoes, pureed (or small pureed can)		

Method

1. Heat oil, fry onions, ginger, and garlic.
2. Add red chilli powder, tomato puree, salt and sugar. Cook on slow fire. Put in blender.
3. Lightly Fry the pieces of tandoori chicken and remove from fat.
4. Remove pan from heat and add tomato sauce (as cooked above) and cook for about 5 minutes.
5. Add buttermilk. Mix it. Cook for 5 minutes.
6. Add the fried chicken. Simmer for 10 minutes or until the flavor of the sauce penetrates.
7. Remove from heat.
8. Sprinkle with roasted ground black cumin seed, garam masala and finely chopped coriander leaves.

Yield:	1 serving
Serving Size:	2 pieces or 1 joint
Calories per serving:	400
Total Fat:	20 g
Cholesterol:	85 mg
Fiber:	-

TANDORI CHICKEN

Ingredients

1 C	low fat yogurt	1/3 C	hungarian paprika
1/4 C	white vinegar	½ T	tomato paste
2-1/4 t	ground cumin	1/4 C	low fat buttermilk or low fat sour cream
1 ½ t	red chili powder	1 t	garlic/ginger paste
1 ½ t	garam masala	2 t	mashed garlic
1 ½ t	salt	2 t	minced ginger
1 T	ground black pepper	1 T	oil

1 medium sized chicken (skinned and cut into pieces)

Method

1. Mix all ingredients well in a large pan.
2. Marinate the chicken for at least 8 hours and preferably overnight, turning the pieces occasionally.
3. Preheat oven to 500°F for at least ½ hour.
4. Put the chicken in a shallow pan. Roast until crusty, about 25 minutes.
5. Turn over and roast 15 minutes more.

Yield:	4 servings
Serving Size:	2 pieces
Calories per serving:	189
Total Fat:	5.5 g
Cholesterol:	75 mg
Fiber:	0.1 g

CHICKEN WITH APRICOTS

Ingredients

1 3-lb	chicken, skinned and cut	2	onions, sliced thin
2	Green chilies	4	tomatoes, chopped
2	Garlic cloves	4	apricots, pits removed, chopped and salted to taste
1 t	cumin seeds	½ C	water
2 T	oil		
2 T	chopped coriander leaves		

Method

1. Grind chilies, garlic and cumin seeds, making into a paste.
2. In a wok, saute onions until golden. Add the chicken pieces and saute over medium heat until chicken is brown, about 15 minutes. Add the masala paste, tomatoes, apricots and salt, plus ½ cup of water. Simmer until meat is tender, 15-20 minutes.

Yield:	4 servings
Serving Size:	2 pieces
Calories per serving:	220
Total Fat:	5.5 g
Cholesterol:	75 mg
Fiber:	2 g

CHICKEN WITH CABBAGE

Ingredients

1 3-pound chicken, skinned and cut	½ t red pepper
1 small cabbage, shredded	1 t salt
2 T oil	2T coriander leaves for garnish
2 onions, chopped fine	
1 T ginger/garlic paste	

Method

1. Boil the chicken in covered water until tender. Remove chicken and reserve stock.
2. Wash and shred the cabbage.
3. In a wok or heavy skillet, heat the oil and lightly saute the onions, garlic, ginger paste and pepper. Stir in the cabbage and the salt. Cook until cabbage is half-way crisp.
4. Add the chicken pieces and the stock and heat through, 5 to 10 minutes.

Yield:	4 servings
Serving Size:	1 bowl
Calories per serving:	230
Total Fat:	5.5 g
Cholesterol:	75 mg
Fiber:	2 g

CHICKEN PALAK
(Spinach)

Ingredients

3-pound chicken, skinned and cut
2 T oil
2 onions, sliced thin
4 garlic cloves, minced
1-inch cinnamon stick
2 t minced fresh ginger
2 t coriander seeds
4 tomatoes, chopped
2 C chopped spinach (or 2 packages frozen cut spinach)

Method

1. Boil the chicken until tender. Remove chicken and reserve stock.
2. Heat the oil in a wok or frying pan, saute the onions and garlic until light brown. Add the minced ginger, coriander seeds, and saute 2 minutes. Add the chicken pieces and saute 5 more minutes, turning chicken on all sides.
3. Add the tomatoes, the spinach, and one half of the chicken stock.
4. Cover and simmer for 20 minutes.

Yield:	4 servings
Serving Size:	1 bowl
Calories per serving:	250
Total Fat:	5.5 g
Cholesterol:	75 mg
Fiber:	3 g

SHRIMP CURRY

Ingredients

shrimps	3 cloves garlic
2 onions	½ t salt
1 tamarind (cleaned and washed)	2 t oil
½ t cumin seeds	1/4 C water
½ t mustard seeds	a few sprigs coriander
2-3 peppercorns	a few curry leaves

Method

1. Except for the shrimp and curry leaves, grind all of the above ingredients together.
2. Heat oil, fry curry leaves, add ground masala and fry well.
3. When brown in color, add shrimp.
4. Lightly fry, adding water and continue cooking until done.

Yield:	1 serving
Serving Size:	1 bowl
Calories per serving:	172
Total Fat:	9 g
Cholesterol:	151 mg
Fiber:	0.7 g

TANDOORI FISH

Ingredients

pomfret, dover sole or halibut, whole		½ t	salt
(singhara or round fish is better for the oven)		½ t	vinegar
½ t	salt	1 t	Ajwain
½ t	chilli powder	½	Lemon (juice)
2 t	ginger	1 t	garam masala
2	cloves garlic	2 t	ginger
½ t	ajwain	2	cloves garlic, a paste
½	lemon	½ t	turmeric
5 T	low fat yogurt	1 T	oil

Method

1. Cut the fish on the belly side and clean the inside. Cut fins and tail, wash well and drain. Give four slits cross-wise evenly spaced on both sides up to the bone. Do not cut bone.
2. Apply salt, chilli powder, ginger, garlic paste and sprinkle with a little of the ajwain powder. Squeeze juice of ½ lemon on top. Leave aside for half an hour.
3. Make a mixture of yogurt, salt, vinegar, ajwain powder, lemon juice, garam masala, ginger garlic paste and turmeric.
4. Marinate prepared fish in this mixture for one hour. Spoon mixture into cuts.
5. Affix to skewers (through mouth and through tail) and cook in moderate oven (350^{0}) for about 20 minutes.
6. Hang to drain the exudate.

Yield:	4 servings
Serving Size:	1 joint
Calories per serving:	160
Total Fat:	6 g
Cholesterol:	-
Fiber:	0.2 g

SALADS

CHICKEN AND BEAN SALAD

Ingredients

1	chicken breast, skinned, cooked and shredded
2	C cooked chick peas (you can use canned)
2	C cooked black-eyed peas
2	carrots, pared and sliced
3	T vegetable oil
2	T vinegar
2	T coriander, chopped
1	t sesame oil
1	t soy sauce (low sodium)
2	t shredded ginger
2	green chillies, chopped
1	small red onion, chopped

Method

Mix all the ingredients together.

Yield:	6 servings
Serving Size:	1 bowl
Calories per serving:	293
Total Fat:	11 g
Cholesterol:	23 mg
Fiber:	8 g

BEAN AND BROCCOLI SALAD

Ingredients

3 C broccoli flowers, cooked crisp
2 C cooked black-eyed peas
1/3 C diced roasted red pepper
2 T olive oil
1 T fresh lemon juice
2 T chopped coriander
2 chopped green chillies (if you like)
salt to taste

Method

Stir all ingredients together in a bowl.

Yield:	2 servings
Serving Size:	1 bowl
Calories per serving:	419
Total Fat:	15 g
Cholesterol:	0 mg
Fiber:	12 g

OAT SALAD

Ingredients

1 C cooked oats
½ C cooked red kidney beans
½ C minced fresh coriander
1/4 C fresh lemon juice
2 scallions, chopped finely
2 T olive oil
2 T minced fresh mint
2 green chillies, cut into small pieces
salt to taste

Method

Stir all ingredients together.

Yield:	4 servings
Serving Size:	1 bowl
Calories per serving:	137
Total Fat:	8 g
Cholesterol:	0 mg
Fiber:	2.5 g

RAITA (Yogurt Salad)

Ingredients

1	large cucumber (about 3/4 pound)
3 C	nonfat yogurt
½ t	freshly ground black pepper
2	small green chilies, chopped
3 T	chopped coriander leaves
1 t	cumin seeds
½ t	garam masalla

Method

1. Wash, peel and grate the cucumber. Squeeze to remove surplus water.
2. In a large bowl, beat the yogurt thoroughly.
3. Mix the cucumber, yogurt, and black pepper together.
4. Transfer the mixture to a serving bowl and sprinkle with chilies and coriander leaves.
5. Heat a griddle and roast the cumin seeds over moderate heat until lightly browned. Then grind the seeds coarsely.
6. On griddle, roast the garam masalla a few seconds and sprinkle it with the cumin over the yogurt as a garnish.

Yield:	6 servings
Serving Size:	1 cup
Calories per serving:	67
Total Fat:	0.2 g
Cholesterol:	2.5 mg
Fiber:	0.2 g

TOMATO RAITA

Ingredients

1 T	vegetable oil
1/8 t	asafetida *(heeng)*
1 t	*chana daal*, a lentil (split yellow pea)
½ T	finely sliced ginger
½ C	finely chopped scallions
1 C	finely chopped tomatoes
3 C	nonfat yogurt
½ t	*garam masalla*, a spice mixture
2 T	chopped green coriander leaves
2	small green chilies, chopped (optional)

Method

1. Heat the oil, drop in the asafetida, and then immediately add the *daal*. Fry 2 minutes. Add the ginger and fry 2 to 3 minutes. Stir in onions and fry 1 minute. Stir in tomatoes and remove from the heat.
2. Beat the yogurt well and stir into the fried tomato mixture. Transfer to a serving bowl.
3. Heat griddle and roast the garam masalla. Stir into the mixture.
4. Garnish with coriander leaves and chilies.

Yield:	6 servings
Serving Size:	1 bowl
Calories per serving:	84
Total Fat:	0.2 g
Cholesterol:	2.5 mg
Fiber:	0.4 g

SPROUTED GREEN DAL RAITA

Ingredients

2T	sprouted green dal (mung)
½ C	nonfat yogurt
½	small, finely chopped onion
½	green chilli (chopped)
	a few coriander leaves
½	t salt
	red chilli powder to taste
1/4 t	roasted and ground cumin seeds

Method

1. Beat the yogurt well until it is of a pouring consistency (by adding water if required).
2. Mix sprouts, onion, chilli, coriander leaves and salt.
3. Garnish with cumin powder and a few coriander leaves.
4. Chill and serve.

Yield:	1 serving
Serving Size:	1 bowl
Calories per serving:	107
Total Fat:	0.2 g
Cholesterol:	2.5 mg
Fiber:	0.6 g

MINT AND PEANUT RAITA

Ingredients

2 T	mint leaves (chopped)
1 T	roasted peanuts
½	green chilli
½ C	nonfat yoghurt
½ t	salt
1/3 t	cumin seeds (roasted and ground)
	a pinch of pepper

Method

1. Wash and grind mint leaves to a fine paste.
2. Pound roasted peanuts and chop chilli.
3. Mix with beaten yogurt of pouring consistency.
4. Season and serve as above.

Yield:	1 serving
Serving Size:	1 bowl
Calories per serving: 160	
Total Fat:	7.2 g
Cholesterol:	2.5 mg
Fiber:	0.6 g

EGGPLANT RAITA

Ingredients

1	large eggplant
3 C	nonfat yogurt
3 ½ T	chopped coriander leaves
½ t	ground black pepper
2	small green chillies, chopped
1 t	roasted cumin seeds
2 t	roasted garam masala

Method

1. Broil eggplant. Cool it. Peel and mash it.
2. In a large bowl, beat the yogurt.
3. Mix together eggplant, yogurt and black pepper together.
4. Transfer to a serving bowl and sprinkle with chillies and coriander leaves.
5. Grind roasted cumin seeds. Sprinkle it with roasted garam masala over yogurt.

Yield:	6 servings
Serving Size:	1 bowl
Calories per serving: 74	
Total Fat:	0.2 g
Cholesterol:	2.5 mg
Fiber:	2 g

DESSERTS

ORANGE SOUFFLE

Ingredients

Cooking spray
1 T sugar
3 T all-purpose flour
3/4 C 1% low-fat milk
1/4 C sugar
2 t grated orange rind
1/4 C fresh orange juice
5 large egg whites (at room temperature)
1/4 t cream of tartar
Dash of salt
2 T sugar
1 t powdered sugar

Method

1. Preheat oven to 375°.
2. Coat a 1 ½- quart souffle dish with cooking spray. Sprinkle with 1 tablespoon sugar. Set aside.
3. Place flour in a small saucepan. Gradually add milk, stirring with a whisk until blended. Add 1/4 cup sugar and rind. Stir well.
4. Bring to a boil over medium heat. Cook 1 minute or until thickened, stirring constantly.
5. Stir in juice and set aside.
6. Beat egg whites, cream of tartar, and salt at high speed with electric mixer until soft peaks form. Gradually add 2 tablespoons sugar, 1 tablespoon at a time, beating until stiff peaks form. Gently fold one-fourth egg white mixture into orange mixture; gently fold in remaining egg white mixture.
7. Spoon into prepared souffle dish and bake at 375° for 40 minutes or until puffy and set.
8. Sprinkle with powdered sugar. Serve immediately.

Yield:	4 servings
Serving Size:	1 cup
Calories per serving: 150	
Total Fat:	1 g
Cholesterol:	10 mg
Fiber:	0.3 g

CAPPUCCINO PUDDING CAKE

Ingredients

1 C	all-purpose flour
2/3 C	sugar
2 T	unsweetened cocoa
2 t	baking powder
½ C	evaporated skim milk
1 t	vegetable oil
1 t	vanilla extract
1/4 C	semisweet chocolate morsels
1 C	firmly packed dark brown sugar
1/4 C	unsweetened cocoa
1 3/4 C	hot water
2	(.77-ounce) envelopes instant cappuccino coffee mix or 1/4 cup other instant flavored coffee mix
9 T	frozen vanilla yogurt

Method

1. Preheat oven to 350°.
2. Combine first 5 ingredients in a 9-inch square baking pan, and stir well.
3. Add milk, oil, and vanilla, stirring until smooth.
4. Stir in chocolate morsels.
5. Combine brown sugar and 1/4 cup cocoa and sprinkle over batter. Combine water and coffee mix, stirring to dissolve.
6. Pour coffee mixture over batter; do not stir.
7. Bake at 350° for 40 minutes or until cake springs back when touched lightly in center.
8. Serve warm with 1 tablespoon frozen yogurt.

Yield:	9 servings
Serving Size:	1 bowl
Calories per serving:	247
Total Fat:	3 g
Cholesterol:	6 mg
Fiber:	0.3 g

KHEER

(Rice Pudding)

Ingredients

½ C rice
2 quarts low-fat (2%) milk
1 T ground cardamon
½ C raisins
2 T sliced almond (skin removed)
½ C sugar
few drops of rose water (optional)

Method

1. Wash the rice and let soak in water for 1 hour.
2. Bring the milk to a boil and add the rice. Stir gently until the mixture thickens a bit, then reduce heat.
3. Add the ground cardamon, raisins and sugar, and the rose water, if used.
4. Stir gently a few minutes until the mixture gets thick and creamy.
5. Add almonds and serve.

Yield:	6 servings
Serving Size:	1 cup
Calories per serving:	240
Total Fat:	4.7 g
Cholesterol:	20 mg
Fiber:	-

SEWIAN KHEER

Ingredients

2 T	almonds
3 T	milk (2%)
2 Quarts	milk
½ C	roasted sewian
½ C	sugar
1 drop	drop kewra essence (optional)
2	pistachio nuts (optional)

Method

1. Blanch the almonds. Remove skin and grind almonds to a fine paste with 3 T milk.
2. Boil the 2 quarts of milk for 10 minutes.
3. Add almonds' paste and boil again.
4. Add the sewian to above and cook on slow fire until they become tender and the mixture thickens to an even consistency.
5. Add sugar and cook for a few minutes stirring continuously as sewian tends to become lumpy and stick to the bottom of the pan.
6. Remove from the fire. Cool and add kewra.
7. Pour into small plate. Sprinkle with finely shredded pistachios over them, if desired.

Yield:	6 servings
Serving Size:	1 bowl
Calories per serving:	240
Total Fat:	4.7 g
Cholesterol:	20 mg
Fiber:	-

PHIRNI

Ingredients

½ C	rice flour
2 Quarts	milk (2%)
½ C	sugar
2 T	shredded blanched almonds
2 T	shredded blanched pistachio nuts

Method

1. Mix rice flour with 1-2 T cold water, make a paste. Strain the paste through a muslin cloth.
2. Mix the rice paste with the milk. Cook on medium heat and stir until the mixture is of creamy consistency.
3. Remove from the fire, add sugar and stir.
4. Return mixture to the stove and simmer until sugar is fully dissolved. Then bring to full boil for 1 minute.
5. Cool the essence and add half of the shredded blanched almonds and pistachios.
6. Pour the mixture into a bowl.
7. Chill.
8. Decorate the dish with the remaining shredded nuts just before serving.

Yield:	6 servings
Serving Size:	1 bowl
Calories per serving:	240
Total Fat:	4.7 g
Cholesterol:	20 mg
Fiber:	-

APRICOT MOUSSE

Ingredients

1	lb dried apricots
½	C sugar
1/4	C cool whip
½	t vanilla
2	T lemon juice

toasted, flaked brown almonds

Method

1. Soak the apricots in water and lemon juice for 12-24 hours.
2. Simmer until tender.
3. Sieve or liquidize and sweeten with sugar.
4. Fold in with whipped cream. Chill.
5. Spoon into small bowl and top with flaked browned almonds.

Yield:	6 servings
Serving Size:	1 bowl
Calories per serving:	100
Total Fat:	0
Cholesterol:	0
Fiber:	2 g

MANDARIN YOGURT DESSERT

Ingredients

1	bowl cool whip - medium size
4	low-fat orange mandarin yogurt
2	cans mandarin segments

Method

Drain mandarin segments and mix well with yogurt and cool whip.

Yield:	8 servings
Serving Size:	1 bowl
Calories per serving:	225
Total Fat:	2.6 g
Cholesterol:	9 mg
Fiber:	.5 g

TABLE 1. RISK PROFILE

TABLE I	
RISK PROFILE	
For each question select one answer that describes your eating habits.	
A.	What kind of milk do you drink or use in cooking? 1. No milk 2. Skim milk 3. One percent milk 4. Two percent milk 5. Whole milk Points________
B.	How many eggs do you eat? 1. Egg white, egg substitute, no eggs 2. One egg/month 3. Two eggs/week 4. Three to six eggs/week 5. More than six eggs/week Points________
C.	What kind of cheese do you eat most often? 1. No cheese 2. Low fat, low cholesterol cheese 3. Part skim milk cheese, e.g. mozzarella 4. Cheddar, swiss, american, cream cheese 5. "Paneer" (Indian cheese) made from whole milk Points________
D.	What kind of fat do you usually use in cooking? 1. Vegetable oil 2. Margarine 3. Shortening (crisco, etc.) 4. Butter 5. Ghee Points________
E.	What kind of meat do you eat more than three times a week? 1. No meat 2. Fish 3. Chicken, turkey 4. Beef, lamb 5. Pork Points________

F.	How often do you eat the following desserts? 1. No desserts, only fresh fruits 2. Mithai (Indian sweets), cheese cake, or other desserts made from whole milk and butter or ghee/twice a week 3. Above (#2)/three times a week 4. #2 four times a week 5. #2 more than four times a week
G.	Do you eat the following snacks more than three times a week> 1. Fruit or no snacks 2. Air-popped popcorn, low-fat crackers 3. Potato chips/corn chips 4. Cookies 5. Nuts Points______________
H.	Do you eat the following breads more than three times a week? 1. Toast or no bread 2. Chappatis or naan (without ghee or butter) 3. Chappatis (with ghee or butter) 4. Croissant 5. Purees/parantha Points______________
I.	How often do you eat pizza? 1. Never 2. One to two times a week 3. Two to three times a week 4. Four times a week 5. More than five times a week Points______________
J.	Which frozen dessert do you eat more than three times a week? 1. None 2. Sherbert 3. Low-fat frozen yoghurt 4. Ice cream 5. "Mithai" (Indian sweets, e.g. Kulfi) Points______________

K.	Do you eat the following Indian snacks more than three times a week? 1. Never 2. Pakora 3. Dalhmoth 4. Mathi 5. Samosa/Kachori Points________________
L.	How often do you add salt to your food at the table? 1. Never 2. Occasionally 3. Frequently 4. Always Points________________
	TOTAL POINTS:
	Interpretation of Points 0-15 Excellent dietary habits 15-30 Very good dietary habits, need few dietary modifications 30-40 Good dietary habits, need few dietary modifications 40-50 Fair dietary habits - need major dietary modifications 50-60 Poor dietary habits - need major dietary modification

TABLE II. SATURATED FATS

TABLE II	
SATURATED FATS	
High Sources	Low Sources
Butterfat	Safflower oil
Lard	Sunflower oil
Coconut oil	Soybean oil
Ghee	Sesame oil
Lamb	Cottonseed oil
Beef	Corn oil
Pork	seeds
Cheddar cheese	Almonds
Egg yolk	Walnuts
Cream	Avocado
Chocolate	Olives
Mithai (Indian Sweets)	Vegetables
	Fruits
	Cereals
	Bread

TABLE III. CHOLESTEROL

TABLE III	
CHOLESTEROL	
High Sources	Low Sources
(Only found in animal products) Egg yolk Organ meats Lard Meat Poultry (especially the skin) Shrimp Oysters Lobster Whole milk Cream Butter Ghee	Beverages Sugars Margarine Vegetable oils Fruits Vegetables Grain products Skim milk Egg White Nuts Avocado Olives

TABLE IV. FIBER

TABLE IV

FIBER

High Sources	Low Sources
Bran	Beverages
Whole grain products	Sugars
Fresh fruits and vegetables	Fats and oils
Seeds	Refined grain products
Nuts	Fish
Crunchy peanut butter	Poultry
Legumes	Eggs
	Milk and milk products

TABLE V. FOODS WITH 3 GRAMS OR MORE OF FIBER

TABLE V		
FOODS WITH 3 GRAMS OR MORE OF FIBER		
1.	Bran cereal	½ cup
2.	Wheat germ	3 Tb
3.	Bean & peas (kidney, black-eye)	1/3 cup
4.	Corn	½ cup
5.	Lima beans	½ cup
6.	Squash	½ cup
7.	Blackberries/blueberries	3/4 cup
8.	Pomagranate	½ cup
9.	Raspberries	1 cup
10.	Strawberries	1 1/4 cup
11.	Dried Fruits	
	Apricots	7 halves
	Prunes	3 medium
	Figs	1 ½
	Apples	4 rings
12.	All vegetables (2-3 g carbohydrates)	½ cup

Suggestions for increasing fiber in the diet

1. Add oat bran flour to chappatis.
2. Eat fresh fruits everyday.
3. Eat dals (pulses, legumes) more frequently.
4. Use oatmeal frequently - breakfast, salads, soups, main dishes.

It is recommended that we consume about 25-35 grams of fiber per day.

TABLE VI. SALT

TABLE VI	
SALT	
High Sources	Low Sources
Table salt Seasoning salts Salty condiments and sauces Monosodium glutamate (MSG) Baking soda Meat tenderizer Cured meats Processed cheese Many convenience foods Canned foods Dalmoth Mathi	Beverages Sugars Fats and oils Salt free cereals Fresh fruits Fresh vegetables

Foods with 400 mg or More of Sodium		
1.	Sauerkraut	
2.	Tomato/vegetable juice	
3.	Luncheon meats	
4.	Sausages	
5.	Frankfurter, turkey or chicken, beef or pork	
6.	All regular cheeses	
7.	Diet cheeses	
8.	Salad dressing (reduced calorie)	
9.	Bouillion	
10.	Pickles	
11.	Soy Sauce	
12.	Pizza	
13.	Chow mein	
14.	Macaroni and cheese	

TABLE VII.
CALORIES, FATS, AND FIBER CONTENT OF SOME FAVORITE FOODS EATEN BY ASIAN AMERICANS

TABLE VII				
CALORIES, FAT & FIBER CONTENT OF SOME FAVORITE FOODS EATEN BY ASIAN AMERICANS				
Food	Amount	Calories	Fat g	Fiber g
Chappati	1 (5" diameter) without butter	80	-	1
Parantha (plain)	1 (medium size)	150	21	1.3
Parantha (potato)	1 (medium)	200	21	2.5
Parantha (cauliflower)	1 (medium)	175	21	3.1
Parantha (radish)	1 (medium)	160	21	3.1
Poori	1 (medium)	100	4	0.3
Katchorie	1	210	33	0.1
Bhatura	1	100	2.5	0.1
Sambhar	1 bowl	164	7.5	1.7
Kala Chana	1 bowl	346	17.8	2.6
Seekh Kabab	1 (4" length)	50	2	0.1
Shami Kabab	1	130	8	0.5
Butter Chicken	1 joint	657	23	2.1
Matar Paneer	1 bowl	406	26	5.3
Carrot halwa	1 small bowl	495	27	2
Suji halwa	1 small bowl	376	23	0.1
Kulfi	1 small moule	322	15	-
Onion pakora	1 medium moule	273	14	0.9
Cauliflower pakora	1 medium	249	15	1.4
Spinach pakora	2	235	14	0.6
Potato pakora	made from 1 potato	304	14	0.7
Paneer Pakora	4 to 5	358	25	0.7
Vegetable Samosa	1 small	150	11	1
Keema Samosa	1 small	200	20	0.1
Mathri	1	102	9	0.1
Gujia	1	200	7.5	0.2
Masala vada	1	80	3	0.3
Dahi Vada	1	105	5	0.1
Coconut Chutney	2T	73	6	0.6
Burfi (plain)	2 pieces	283	13.5	-
Burfi (coconut)	2 pieces	472	29	1.6
Burfi (cashewnut)	2 pieces	166	8	0.2
Burfi (besan)	2 pieces	265	14	0.3
Besan ladoo	2	308	19	0.3
Rava ladoo (nuts)	2	189	11	0.1
Till ladoos	2	157	7.2	0.5
Gulab Jamun (milk powder)	2	161	5	-
Gulab Jamun (khoya)	2	197	11	-
Chum chum	1	124	5	-
Rasmalai	1	300	16	-

TABLE VIII.
NUTRIENT CONTENT OF FOODS
FREQUENTLY EATEN BY
ASIAN AMERICANS FROM FAST FOOD
RESTAURANTS

TABLE VIII						
NUTRIENT CONTENT OF FOODS FREQUENTLY EATEN BY ASIAN AMERICANS FROM FAST FOOD RESTAURANTS						
Food	Serving size	Calories	Total Fat g	Cholesterol mg	Fiber g	Sodium mg
PIZZA						
Domino						
Cheese	1 slice	180	5	10	-	500
Veggie pizza	1 slice	195	6.5	12.5	-	545
Pepperoni	1 slice	205	7.5	17.5	-	595
PIZZA HUT						
Hand tossed						
Cheese	1 slice	259	10	27.5	-	638
Pepperoni	1 slice	259	11.5	25	-	634
Supreme	1 slice	270	13	27.5	-	735
Pan Pizza						
Cheese	1 slice	246	9	17	-	470
Pepperoni	1 slice	206	11	23	-	568
Supreme	1 slice	230	11	21	-	664
Thin'n'crispy						
Cheese	1 slice	199	8.5	16.5	-	434
Pepperoni	1 slice	207	10	23	-	493
Supreme	1 slice	230	11	21	-	664
BURGER KING						
Apple pie	1	311	14	24	-	412
Cheese burger	1	318	15	50	-	661
Chicken tenders	1 order	236	13	38	-	541
French fries	1 order	341	20	21	-	241
KENTUCKY FRIED CHICKEN						
Breast, extra crispy	1	365	23	80	-	640
Breast, hot & spicy	1	382	26	84	-	905
Chicken sandwich	1	169	10	18	1	331
Chicken nuggets	6	284	18	66	-	865
Coleslaw	1 order	114	6	4	-	177
Corn-on-the-cob	1	90	2	-	1	11
Drumstick, extra crispy	1	205	14	72	-	292
Drumstick, hot & spicy	1	207	14	75	-	406
French Fries	1 order	244	12	2	1	139
Hot wings	6	471	33	150	-	1230
Food	Serving size	Calories	Total Fat g	Cholesterol mg	Fiber g	Sodium mg

Rotisserie Gold						
Chicken						
Dark Quarter (with	1	333	23.7	163	-	980
skin)						
Dark Quarter	1	217	12.2	128	-	772
(without skin)						
McDonald's						
Apple Bran Muffin	1	180	-	-	-	200
Big Mac	1	500	26	100	1	890
Biscuit with bacon,	1	440	26.4	253	1	1215
egg, and cheese						
Biscuit with sausage	1	505	33	260	1	1210
& egg						
Chicken McNuggets	6	270	15	55	-	580
Chocolate Chip	pieces					
Cookies		330	15	4	-	280
Egg McMuffin	1 box	290	11.2	226	-	710
French Fries	1					
Small		220	12	-	1	110
Medium	1 order	320	17	-	1	150
Large	1 order	400	21.6	-	1	200
Hamburger	1 order	255	9	37	-	490
Hash Browns	1	130	7.3	-	-	330
Pie, apple	1 order	260	148	6	-	240
Shake	1					
Chocolate		320	1.7	10	-	240
Strawberry	1	320	1.3	10	-	170
Vanilla	1	230	1.0	33		35
	1					
Taco Bell						
Burrito, bean	1	381	14	9	1	1148
Burrito, chicken	1	334	12	52	-	880
Burrito, combo	1	407	16	33	-	1136
Burrito, supreme	1	383	18	47	-	893
Mexican Pizza	1	575	37	52	-	1031
Nachos	1 order	346	18	9	-	399
Nacho supreme	1 order	367	27	18	-	471

TABLE IX.
CALORIES, FAT AND CHOLESTEROL CONTENT OF SELECTED FOODS

TABLE IX: CALORIES, FAT, AND CHOLESTEROL CONTENT OF SELECTED FOODS				
ITEM	**PORTION**	**CALORIES**	**FAT GRAMS**	**CHOLESTEROL mg**
BEVERAGES: Alcoholic				
Beer				
Regular	12 fl. oz.	146	0.0	0
Light, Budweiser	12 fl. oz.	110	0.0	0
Champagne	6 fl. oz.	135	0.0	0
Gin	6 fl. oz.	87	0.0	0
80 proof				
Pina colada	1-1/2 fl. oz.			
Rum	6 fl. oz.	103	0.0	0
80 proof		262	2.7	0
Sherry, medium	1-1/2 fl. oz.			
Vodka	6 fl. oz.	103	0.0	0
80 proof		210	0.0	0
Whiskey	1-1/2 fl. oz.			
80 proof		103	0.0	0
Wine, dessert	1-1/2 fl. oz.			
(18.8% alcohol)		103	0.0	0
Dry				
Sweet	6 fl. oz.	224	0.0	0
	6 fl. oz.	272	0.0	0
BEVERAGES: Nonalcoholic				
Coca-Cola	12 fl. oz.	140	0.0	0
Coffee, regular brewed	6 fl. oz.	4	0.0	0
Coffee, Instant Decaffeinated	6 fl. oz.	11	0.0	0
Fruit punch, canned	6 fl. oz.	4	0.0	0
Juice				
Apple, canned or bottled	1 cup	117	0.0	0
Blackberry,	½ cup	58	0.1	0
unsweetened, canned				
Cranberry	½ cup	45	0.7	0
Cranberry/apple, w/vit. C	½ cup	75	0.1	0
Grape, canned or bottled	½ cup	82	0.0	0
Grape, sparkling				
Red, Welch's	½ cup	77	0.1	0
Grapefruit, canned				
Unsweetened	6 fl. oz.	117	0.0	0
Sweetened	½ cup	47	0.1	0
Orange, fresh	½ cup	58	0.1	0
Orange/grape canned	½ cup	56	0.2	0
Pineapple/grapefruit	½ cup	53	0.1	0
Pineapple/orange	½ cup	67	0.0	0
Pineapple, unsweetened,	½ cup	67	0.1	0
Canned	½ cup	70	0.1	0
Prune, canned or bottled				
	½ cup	91	0.0	0

CALORIES, FAT, AND CHOLESTEROL CONTENT OF SELECTED FOODS				
ITEM	**PORTION**	**CALORIES**	**FAT GRAMS**	**CHOLESTEROL mg**
BEVERAGES: Nonalcoholic				
Tomato, regular				
Canned/bottled	½ cup	21	0.1	0
Vegetable, Cocktail, canned				
V-8, no salt	½ cup	23	0.1	0
Kool-Aid, cherry	½ cup	24	0.1	-
Lemonade,	1 cup	88	0.0	0
Regular, frozen, dilute				
Pink, prepared	1 cup	99	0.0	0
Country Time	1 cup	94	0.0	0
Nectar, canned				
Apricot				
Peach, 40% Fruit	½ cup	70	0.1	0
Seltzer, unsweetened	½ cup	67	0.2	0
Soda	12 fl. oz.	0	0.0	0
Club				
Orange	12 fl. oz.	0	0.0	0
Tang, orange, prepared	12 fl. oz.	170	0.0	0
Tea, brewed	1 cup	119	0.0	0
Tea, instant, prepared	6 fl. oz.	2	0.0	0
Quinine water				
BREADS/BREADSTUFFS				
Bagels				
Plain	1	161	1.5	-
Lenders	1	179	0.4	0
Biscuits				
Buttermilk	1	60	1.5	-
Breads				
7 Grain	1 slice	80	0.4	3
Brown, Boston, canned	1 slice	93	0.5	0
French	1 slice	70	1.0	0
Du Jour	1 slice	111	4.3	1
Garlic	1 slice	147	1.1	
Pita				
Plain	1 slice	76	0.4	0
Pumpernickel	1 slice	66	0.7	0
Raisin	1 slice	61	0.8	1
Wheat				
Regular	1 slice	95	1.5	-
Pepperidge Farm	1 slice	60	1.0	0
White				
Wonder	1 slice	198	8.9	48

CALORIES, FAT, AND CHOLESTEROL CONTENT OF SELECTED FOODS				
ITEM	**PORTION**	**CALORIES**	**FAT GRAMS**	**CHOLESTEROL mg**
BREADS/ BREADSTUFFS				
Breads, Sweetened				
Coffeecake				
Danish	2 oz.	198	8.9	48
Apple				
Cheese	1	335	15.9	19
Donut	1	353	24.6	20
Muffins				
Plain				
Cinnamon Raisin-Chip				
Pepperidge Farm	1	150	2.0	-
Thomas'	1	130	1.4	0
Rolls				
Croissant				
Regular				
Hamburger bun	1	272	17.3	47
Hot dog bun	1	136	3.4	13
Tortilla	1	136	3.4	13
BREAKFAST FOODS				
Cereal				
All Bran, Kellogg's	1/3 cup	69	1.0	0
Apple Jacks	1 cup	111	0.6	0
Cherrios, plain	1 cup	89	1.5	0
Honey Nut	1 cup	125	0.7	0
Cinnamon Toast Crunch	1 cup	160	4.0	0
Corn Flakes, Kellogg's				
Plain	1 cup	88	0.1	0
Sugar Frosted	1 cup	133	0.1	0
Farina, cooked	1 cup	116	0.2	0
Granola				
Cinnamon/raisin	½ cup	160	5.6	0
Grape-nuts	1/3 cup	135	0.2	0
Oat Bran O's				
Plain, Healthy Valley	1 cup	120	2.7	0
Fruit-n-Nut	1 cup	120	2.7	0
Oatmeal, cooked	1 cup	145	2.3	0
Oatmeal, instant	1 cup	94	2.0	0
Rice, puffed	1 cup	114	0.1	0
Rice Krispies	1 cup	112	0.2	0
Special K, Kellogg's	1 cup	83	0.1	0
Sugar Frosted Flakes, Kellogg's	1 cup	133	0.1	0
Wheaties	1 cup	99	0.5	0

CALORIES, FAT, AND CHOLESTEROL CONTENT OF SELECTED FOODS				
ITEM	**PORTION**	**CALORIES**	**FAT GRAMS**	**CHOLESTEROL mg**
BREAKFAST FOODS				
Pancakes				
Blueberry, Aunt Jemima	2	136	1.0	-
Buttermilk	2	329	10.7	108
Prepared				
Plain	2 (4" ea.)	316	10.9	117
Mix, Aunt Jemima	1 oz.	61	2.3	-
Waffles				
Apple cinnamon	1	90	30	-
Aunt Jemima				
Belgian, frozen	1 (1.5 oz.)	120	4.0	5
CANDY				
Almond Joy	1.76 oz. Bar	142	7.9	-
Chocolate-coated	1 oz.	161	12.4	0
Sugar-coated	1 oz.	129	5.3	0
Baby Ruth	1.8 oz. Bar	145	6.1	0
Chocolate bar, plain	1 oz.			
Hershey	1 oz.	153	8.8	7
Nestle's		159	7.9	6
Chocolate bar w/nuts	1 oz.			
w/almonds, Cadbury	1 oz.	153	8.9	-
Hershey	1 oz.	159	10	8
Nestle's Crunch		149	7.9	6
COOKIES				
Brownie, w/o nuts	1			
Regular	1	243	10.1	10
Large, Hostess		243	9.6	17
Brownie w/nuts	1			
Regular	1.2 oz.	263	16.4	81
Fudge-n-Nut, Almost Home		160	7.0	-
Chocolate Chip	1			
Homemade	1	69	4.6	7
Pepperidge Farm	1	50	2.7	-
Gingersnap, small		36	1.3	3
CRACKERS				
	1 oz.			
Cheese Nips	1 oz.	132	5.7	-
Cheese & peanut butter	½ oz.	132	5.7	-
Nabisco	1 oz.	120	2.0	0
Triscuit		142	4.7	0
Wheat Thins	1 oz.			
Regular		142	6.0	0

CALORIES, FAT, AND CHOLESTEROL CONTENT OF SELECTED FOODS				
ITEM	**PORTION**	**CALORIES**	**FAT GRAMS**	**CHOLESTEROLmg**
DAIRY/DAIRY PRODUCTS				
Cheese Whiz, Kraft				
Swiss				
Regular	1 oz.	77	5.8	18
Kraft	1 oz.	107	7.8	26
Swiss, Lite	1 oz.	92	7.0	23
Lifetime, non-fat				
Weight Watchers, skim,	1 oz.	40	0.0	3
semisoft	1 oz.	80	5.2	-
Milk & Milk Beverages				
Buttermilk, whole	1 cup	98	2.1	10
Buttermilk, low fat, low salt,				
friendship	1 cup	120	4.0	-
Condensed, sweetened,				
canned	2 tbl.	123	3.3	13
Cream, Half & Half	2 tbl.	39	3.5	11
Cream, heavy				
Whipped	2 tbl.	51	5.5	20
Unwhipped	2 tbl.	103	11.0	41
Cream, light (coffee/table)	1 tbl.	29	2.9	10
Cream, light (whipping)				
Whipped	2 tbl.	44	4.6	17
Unwhipped	2 tbl.	87	9.2	33
Cream, sour	2 tbl.	62	6.0	13
Half & Half	2 tbl.	41	3.6	11
Milk, chocolate, whole	1 cup	208	8.5	30
Milk, whole, 3.3% fat	1 cup	149	8.1	34
Milk, Low-fat	1 cup	102	2.5	10
1% fat	1 cup	122	4.7	20
2% fat	1 cup	86	0.4	5
Milk, skim				
Milk, non-fat	1/4 cup	109	0.2	6
Dry, Instant Carnation	1 cup	260	0.5	13
Milkshake				
Thick, frosty, Quik, Nestle's	1 cup	282	6.4	24
Chocolate	1 cup	622	27.6	-
Strawberry	2 tbl.	36	0.5	0
	2 tbl.	41	0.0	0
Yogurt				
Plain				
Regular	1 cup	138	7.4	30
Low-fat	1 cup	143	3.5	14
Non-fat. Flavored	1 cup	127	0.4	5
Coffee or vanilla, low-fat				
Fruit varieties, low-fat	1 cup	193	2.8	11
	1 cup	225	2.6	9

CALORIES, FAT, AND CHOLESTEROL CONTENT OF SELECTED FOODS				
ITEM	**PORTION**	**CALORIES**	**FAT GRAMS**	**CHOLESTEROL mg**
DESSERTS				
Angel Food				
Banana, Sara Lee	2 oz.	200	7.8	-
Carrot				
Homemade, prepared	2 oz.	203	11.9	32
Pepperidge Farm	2 oz.	204	11.6	-
Cheesecake, Regular	2 oz.	188	13.7	64
Cheesecake, frozen	2 oz.	167	10.9	-
Chocolate, Commercial				
Loaf, non-fat, Entenmann's	2 oz.	140	0.0	0
Fruit cake, light homemade	2 oz.	221	9.4	0
German chocolate layer	2 oz.	222	12.3	-
Chocolate meringue	3 oz.	180	6.8	55
Coconut custard	3 oz.	171	9.8	82
Puddings				
Rice, w/raisins	½ cup	193	4.0	15
Tapioca	½ cup	111	4.1	80
Vanilla, instant prepared, From mix, Jello	½ cup	76	2.0	-
Other Desserts				
Baklava, homemade	1 oz.	112	8.2	20
Eclair				
Whipped cream filling & Chocolate icing	1	296	25.0	-
Trifle, chocolate	1	69	1.5	1
EGGS, EGG DISHES & EGG SUBSTITUTES				
Eggs				
White only, fresh, raw	1	16	0.0	0
Yolk only, fresh raw	1	61	5.2	218
Fried	1	54	6.8	207
Hard cooked	1	78	5.3	213
Poached, in salt water	1	75	5.0	212
Scrambled	1	103	7.6	218
Soft cooked	1	78	5.3	213
Egg Substitutes				
Egg Beaters, Fleischmann's	1/4 cup	30	0.0	0
FAST FOODS				
Arby's				
Apple turnover	1 serv.	310	21.0	0
Chicken breast				
Roasted	1 serv.	254	7.0	196
Sandwich	1 serv.	592	27.0	57

CALORIES, FAT, AND CHOLESTEROL CONTENT OF SELECTED FOODS				
ITEM	**PORTION**	**CALORIES**	**FAT GRAMS**	**CHOLESTEROL mg**
FAST FOODS				
Hardees				
Apple Turnover	1 serv.	282	14.0	-
Big country breakfast w/bacon	1 serv.	754	12.0	-
Cheeseburger				
Bacon	1 serv.	556	33.0	-
Regular	1 serv.	309	13.0	-
Biscuit				
Cinnamon/raisin	1 serv.	276	16	-
Sausage/egg	1 serv.	52	35.0	-
Hamburger	1 serv.	276	15	-
Milkshake	11 fl. oz.	161	9.0	-
Salad, side	1 serv.	21	0.0	0
The Lean	1 serv.	410	18	-
Kentucky Fried Chicken				
Bake bean	1 serv.	105	1.2	0
Bread, original, side order	1	276	17.3	96
Breast, center				
Original	1 serv.	257	13.7	93
Light/Crispy	1	220	11.9	-
Extra-crispy	1 serv.	353	20.9	93
Chicken nuggets	1 serv.	46	2.9	12
Coleslaw	1 serv.	103	5.7	4
Corn-on-the-cob	1 serv.	176	3.1	0
Drumstick				
Light/Crispy	1 serv.	121	7.0	-
Extra-crispy	1 serv.	173	3.1	0
French Fries	1 serv.	268	12.8	2
Gravy, Chicken	1 serv.	59	3.7	2
Potatoes, Mashed	1 serv.	59	0.6	0
Roll	1 serv.	269	13.6	-
Side Breast, extra-crispy	1 serv.	354	23.7	66
Thigh				
Original	1 serv.	278	19.2	122
Light/Crispy	1 serv.	246	16.7	-
Extra-crispy	1 serv.	371	26.3	121
Wing				
Extra-crispy	1 serv.	218	15.6	63
McDonalds				
Big Mac	1 serv.	570	35.0	83

CALORIES, FAT, AND CHOLESTEROL CONTENT OF SELECTED FOODS				
ITEM	**PORTION**	**CALORIES**	**FAT GRAMS**	**CHOLESTEROL mg**
FAST FOODS				
McDonalds				
Biscuit				
With spread	1 serv.	287	18.2	9
With bacon/egg/cheese	1 serv.	483	31.5	262
With sausage	1 serv.	467	30.9	48
With sausage/egg	1 serv.	585	39.7	285
Danish				
Apple	1 serv.	389	17.9	26
Cheese, iced	1 serv.	395	21.7	48
Cheeseburger	1 serv.	315	15.8	40
Chicken McNuggetts	4 oz.	323	21.3	73
Cookies				
Chocolaty chip	1 serv.	337	16.0	18
McDonaldland	1 serv.	309	10.8	10
Dressings				
French, reduced calorie	½ oz.	40	1.9	0
Egg McMuffin	1 serv.	337	15.5	257
Filet-o-Fish	1 serv.	432	25.6	45
French Fries				
Regular	1 serv.	220	11.4	9
Large	1 serv.	100	21.6	16
Hamburger	1 serv.	264	11.3	29
Ice cream cone	1 serv.	182	5.1	23
McChicken sandwich	1 serv.	490	28.6	43
McD.L.T.	1 serv.	681	43.9	101
McLean deluxe	1 serv.	320	10.00	60
Muffin				
Apple bran	1 serv.	190	0	0.0
English Muffin w/butter	1 serv.	186	5.3	15
Pancake w/butter & syrup	1 serv.	501	10.3	47
Pie				
Apple	1 serv.	253	14.2	13
Cherry	1 serv.	257	13.5	13
Potatoes, hash brown	1 serv.	125	7.0	50.4
Sausage	1 serv.	206	18.3	38
Sausage McMuffin				
Regular	1 serv.	423	26.0	58
With egg	1 serv.	513	32.6	285
Scrambled Eggs	1 serv.	180	13.0	514
Shake				
Chocolate	1 serv.	381	8.7	29
Strawberry	1 serv.	363	8.7	32
Vanilla	1 serv.	352	8.4	32

CALORIES, FAT, AND CHOLESTEROL CONTENT OF SELECTED FOODS				
ITEM	**PORTION**	**CALORIES**	**FAT GRAMS**	**CHOLESTEROL mg**
Taco Bell				
Burrito				
Bean	1 serv.	340	11.7	-
Beef	1 serv.	464	20.9	-
Combination	1 serv.	403	15.9	-
Enchirito	1 serv.	449	20.6	-
Pintos 'N' Cheese	1 serv.	167	5.0	-
Taco	1 serv.	183	7.9	-
Tostada				
Regular	1 serv.	177	5.9	-
Beefy	1 serv.	289	14.9	-
FATS AND OILS				
Butter				
Stick	1 tb.	102	11.5	31
Whipped	1 tb.	68	7.7	21
Butter, imitation				
Butter buds, dry powder	1 tb.	18	0.0	1
Butter buds, prepared	1 tb.	6	0.0	0
Molly McButter	1 tb.	24	0.0	0
Chicken Fat	1 tb.	115	12.8	11
Margarine				
Regular	1 tb.	101	11.4	0
Fleishchmann's	1 tb.	100	11.2	-
Mrs. Filbert's, 100% veg.	1 tb.	100	11	0
Mazola	1 tb.	99	11.2	0
Parkay Spread, 70% veg.	1 tb.	88	9.7	0
Promise Stick	1 tb.	90	10.0	0
Promise, soft	1 tb.	100	11.2	0
Margarine, light or diet, stick	1 tb.	50	5.6	0
Fleischmann's, Extra light	1 tb.	50	6.0	0
Fleischmann's, light	1 tb.	81	8.1	0
Oil, all types	1 tb.	121	13.6	0
Pam, spray	1 spray	2	0.2	0
FISH AND SHELLFISH				
Abalone, raw	3 oz.	89	0.6	72
Bass				
Black Sea, raw	3 oz.	97	3.1	58
Stripped, raw	3 oz.	82	2.0	68
Crab				
Blue, canned, drained	3 oz.	84	1.0	76
Blue, cooked	3 oz.	87	1.5	85
Fish sticks, frozen, cooked	1	76	3.4	31

CALORIES, FAT, AND CHOLESTEROL CONTENT OF SELECTED FOODS				
ITEM	**PORTION**	**CALORIES**	**FAT GRAMS**	**CHOLESTEROL mg**
FISH AND SHELLFISH				
Fish cake, frozen, cooked	3 oz.	231	10.4	95
Halibut, cooked	3 oz.	119	2.5	35
Mackerel				
Atlantic, cooked	3 oz.	223	15.1	64
Monkfish, raw	3 oz.	65	1.3	21
Perch, ocean				
Raw	3 oz.	80	1.4	36
Cooked	3 oz.	103	1.8	46
Rockfish, cooked	3 oz.	103	1.7	37
Salmon				
Atlantic, raw	3 oz.	121	5.4	47
Pink, canned	3 oz.	118	5.1	-
Smoke (Lox)	3 oz.	100	3.7	20
Sockeye, canned	3 oz.	130	6.2	37
Sadine				
Atlantic, canned in oil	3 ½ oz.	200	11.0	17
Shrimp				
Fried, breaded	3 oz.	206	10.4	151
Steamed, large	3 oz.	84	0.9	151
Sole				
Raw	3 oz.	77	1.0	41
Cooked	3 oz.	100	1.3	58
Tuna, canned				
Light, in oil, drained	3 oz.	225	19.1	36
Light, in water drained	3 oz.	90	1.5	36
FRUITS				
Apples				
Fresh	1	81	0.0	0
Dried	1	19	0.0	0
Applesauce				
Canned, unsweetened	½ cup	52	0.0	0
Canned, sweetened	½ cup	97	0.0	0
Apricots				
Fresh	1	18	0.0	0
Canned w/skin, heavy syrup	½ cup	114	0.0	0
Dried, uncooked	1	17	0.0	0
Avocado, fresh				
California	1	306	29.8	0
Florida	1	339	26.7	0
Banana, fresh	1	109	0.0	0
Blackberries				
Fresh	½ cup	37	0.0	0
Frozen, unsweetened Not thawed	½ cup	48	0.0	0
Blueberries				
Fresh	½ cup	41	0.0	0
Frozen, unsweetened	½ cup	42	0.0	0

CALORIES, FAT, AND CHOLESTEROL CONTENT OF SELECTED FOODS				
ITEM	**PORTION**	**CALORIES**	**FAT GRAMS**	**CHOLESTEROL mg**
FRUITS				
Cantaloupe, fresh	1/4 cup	45	0.0	0
Cherries, fresh				
Sour, red w/o pits	½ cup	39	0.0	0
Sweet	½ cup	52	0.0	0
Cherries, canned				
Sour, red, water, packed	½ cup	44	0.0	0
Sour, red, heavy syrup	½ cup	127	0.0	0
Sweet, water-packed	½ cup	62	0.0	0
Sweet, heavy syrup	½ cup	107	0.2	0
Cherries, Maraschino	½ cup	162	0.0	0
Coconut				
Fresh	1 whole	1,349	127.7	0
Shredded, dried, sweetened	1 ½ cup	232	16.4	0
Crabapples, fresh	1 each	23	0.0	0
Cranberries, fresh	½ cup	23	0.0	0
Cranberry sauce, canned, Sweetened	½ cup	209	0.0	0
Currants, fresh				
Black, European	½ cup	35	0.0	0
Red or white	½ cup	31	0.0	0
Figs				
Fresh, medium	1	37	0.0	0
Dried	1	48	0.0	0
Canned, light syrup	½ cup	87	0.0	0
Fruit Cocktail, canned				
Juice packed	½ cup	57	0.0	0
In heavy syrup	½ cup	93	0.0	0
Fruit Salad, canned				
Water packed	½ cup	37	0.0	0
Heavy syrup	½ cup	93	0.0	0
Grapefruit				
Fresh	1	77	0.0	0
Canned, sweetened	½ cup	76	0.0	0
Grapes, fresh				
Concord	½ cup	29	0.0	0
Emperor	½ cup	57	0.0	0
Thompson	½ cup	57	0.0	0
Guavas, common fresh	1	41	0.0	0
Honeydew, fresh cubed	½ cup	30	0.0	0
Kiwi fruit	1	44	0.0	0
Kumquat, fresh	1	12	0.0	0
Lemons, fresh				
With peel	1	22	0.0	0
Without peel	1	16	0.0	0
Plum				
Fresh	1	35	0.0	0
Purple, canned, in heavy syrup	½ cup	115	0.0	0

CALORIES, FAT, AND CHOLESTEROL CONTENT OF SELECTED FOODS				
ITEM	**PORTION**	**CALORIES**	**FAT GRAMS**	**CHOLESTEROL mg**
FRUITS				
Pomegranate pulp, fresh	1	104	0.0	0
Prunes				
Dried, uncooked	1 med	20	0.0	0
Cooked, no sugar	½ cup	134	0.0	0
Quince, fresh	1	52	0.0	0
Raisins				
Black	½ cup	217	0.0	0
Golden	½ cup	219	0.0	0
Raspberries				
Black, fresh	½ cup	33	0.0	0
Red, fresh	½ cup	30	0.0	0
Red, frozen, sweetened	½ cup	129	0.0	0
Rhubarb, cooked, added sugar	½ cup	157	0.0	0
Strawberries				
Fresh	1 cup	45	0.0	0
Frozen, unsweetened	1 cup	52	0.0	0
Tangerines	1	38	0.0	0
Watermelon, fresh, diced	½ cup	26	0.0	0
ICE CREAM, FROZEN YOGURT AND NON-DAIRY FROZEN DESSERTS				
Ice Cream				
Chocolate	½ cup	155	7.2	19
Chocolate cup, Breyers	5 oz.	160	8.0	-
Strawberry	½ cup	116	5.0	16
Vanilla				
10% fat, regular	½ cup	134	7.2	30
16% fat, rich	½ cup	175	11.8	44
Frozen Yogurt				
Low-fat, Colombo	4 fl. oz.	99	2.0	10
Non-fat				
Colombo	4 fl. oz.	95	0.0	0
TCBY	4 fl. oz.	110	1.0	5
Sherbert, lemon	½ cup	104	0.9	0
Sorbet, strawberry	½ cup	71	0.3	0
MEAT				
Brisket, flat, lean, braised	3 oz.	224	13.5	77
Chuck				
Arm, lean, braised	3 oz.	196	8.5	86

CALORIES, FAT, AND CHOLESTEROL CONTENT OF SELECTED FOODS				
ITEM	**PORTION**	**CALORIES**	**FAT GRAMS**	**CHOLESTEROL mg**
MEATS				
Blade, lean, braised	3 oz.	230	13.0	90
Ground				
Extra-lean, boiled	3 oz. patty	218	13.9	71
Lean, broiled	3 oz. patty	231	15.7	74
Rib eye, lean, broiled	3 oz.	191	9.9	68
Round				
Bottom, lean, braised	3 oz.	189	8.2	82
Eye, lean, roasted	3 oz.	156	4.0	77
Tip, lean, roasted	3 oz.	162	6.4	69
Top, lean, broiled	3 oz.	162	5.3	71
Steak, flank, lean, broiled	3 oz.	207	12.7	60
Tenderloin, lean broiled	3 oz.	173	7.9	71
Lamb				
Chop				
Loin, broiled, lean only	3 oz.	160	6.0	44
Loin, broiled, lean & fat	3 oz.	305	25.0	85
Rib				
Cooked, lean only	3 oz.	200	11.0	77
Cooked, lean & fat	3 oz.	307	25.2	84
Shoulder				
Cooked, lean only	3 oz.	173	9.2	74
Cooked, lean & fat	3 oz.	290	23.0	78
Leg, lean, roasted	3 oz.	160	6.0	79
Ham				
Country style, cured, lean	3 oz.	173	10.9	46
Fresh				
Roasted, lean and fat	3 oz.	233	15.1	81
Loin, sirloin, raw				
Lean only	3 oz.	128	5.7	54
Lean and fat	3 oz.	235	19.0	60
Pork				
Boston butt, roasted, lean only	3 oz.	233	15.1	81
Chop, lean				
Rib, lean, braised	3 oz.	230	12.0	0
Veal				
Cubed, for stew, braised, lean only	3 oz.	160	3.7	123
Cutlet, breaded	3 oz.	115	2.3	14
Leg, braised				
Lean only	3 oz.	173	4.3	115
Lean & fat	3 oz.	179	5.4	114

CALORIES, FAT, AND CHOLESTEROL CONTENT OF SELECTED FOODS				
ITEM	**PORTION**	**CALORIES**	**FAT GRAMS**	**CHOLESTEROL mg**
Prepared or Processed Meats				
Bacon, regular				
Canadian, broiled or fried,				
Cured, broiled or drained	1 slice	37	1.7	12
Bacon, imitation	1 slice	43	3.7	6
Bits				
Beef, Sizzlelean	3 oz.	264	25.1	0
Breakfast strips, Sizzlelean	2 strips	70	5.0	-
Beef, corned	1 slice	49	3.9	-
Buddig, lean				
Canned	1 slice	40	2.0	-
Cooked	1 oz.	71	4.2	24
Bologna	1 oz.	71	5.4	28
Beef, Oscar Mayer				
Beef & Pork	1 slice	72	6.7	13
Turkey, Louis Rich	2 oz.	179	16.0	31
Chicken roll, light meat	1 slice	58	4.7	19
Chicken, sliced Buddig	2 oz.	90	4.2	28
Corn dog	1 slice	60	4.0	-
Frankfurter	1	460	18.9	79
Beef, Oscar Mayer				
Pork & beef w/cheese	1	141	13.2	27
Ham Loaf, glazed	2 oz.	185	16.4	39
Ham, chopped, canned	3 oz.	236	14.3	90
Hot Dog	3 oz.	203	16.0	42
Beef				
Chicken	1	176	16.0	34
Pastrami	1	113	8.6	44
Beef				
Turkey	2 oz.	198	16.5	53
^Pate	2 oz.	69	2.9	31
Chicken liver, canned				
Pepperoni, pork and beef	3 oz.	171	11.1	-
Pork, cooked	1 slice	27	2.4	4
Salami	3 oz.	256	21.9	51
Beef				
Pork, dry or hard	2 oz.	142	11.4	37
Sausage	2 oz.	231	19.1	-
Brown 'n' Serve, Jones				
Light, w/rice, Jones	1 link	100	10.0	-
	1 link	70	5.5	-
NUTS, SEEDS & PEANUT BUTTER				
Almonds, raw, natural Blue				
Beechnuts, shelled	1 oz.	165	14.9	0
	1 oz.	163	14.2	0

CALORIES, FAT, AND CHOLESTEROL CONTENT OF SELECTED FOODS				
ITEM	**PORTION**	**CALORIES**	**FAT GRAMS**	**CHOLESTEROL mg**
NUTS, SEEDS & PEANUT BUTTER				
Brazil nuts, dried	2 tb.	115	11.6	0
Cashews				
Dry roasted	2 tb.	98	7.9	0
Oil-roasted, Planters	1 tb.	170	14.0	0
Chestnut, fresh	2 tb.	39	0.4	0
Coconut				
Raw, not packed	2 tb.	35	3.4	0
Dried, sweetened				
Shredded	1 tb.	29	2.1	0
Hazelnuts, shelled whole	2 tb.	107	10.6	0
Macadamia, dried	2 tb.	118	12.4	0
Mixed				
Oil-roasted, no peanuts	2 tb.	111	10.1	0
Roasted w/peanuts	2 tb.	110	10.0	0
Peanuts, roasted				
In shell	1 cup	209	17.7	0
With oil	½ cup	450	35.0	0
Dry roasted, Planters	1 oz.	160	13.9	-
Honey roasted, Planters	1 oz.	170	13.0	0
Peanut Butter				
Chunky	1 tb.	95	8.1	0
Smooth	1 tb.	95	8.3	0
Pecans, shelled, halves	2 tb.	90	9.1	0
Pine, pignolia	2 tb.	103	10.1	0
Pistachio, dry roasted	2 tb.	92	7.7	0
Poppy seeds	2 tb.	94	7.8	0
Pumpkin seed kernels, dry	2 tb.	93	7.9	0
Sesame seeds, dry, whole	2 tb.	103	8.9	0
Sunflower seeds	2 tb.	103	8.9	0
Trail mix, w/coconut	1 oz.	143	11.0	0
Walnuts, Black	2 tb.	95	8.8	0
Persian or English shelled, halves	2 tb.	80	7.7	0
PASTA & NOODLES				
Macaroni, regular				
Cooked	1 cup	197	0.9	0
Cooked, al dente	1 cup	155	0.6	0
Spirals, cooked	1 cup	189	0.9	0
Manicotti, cheese Stouffer's	8 oz.	234	10.9	34

CALORIES, FAT, AND CHOLESTEROL CONTENT OF SELECTED FOODS				
ITEM	**PORTION**	**CALORIES**	**FAT GRAMS**	**CHOLESTEROL mg**
PASTA & NOODLES				
Noodles, chow mein canned	1 cup	237	13.8	0
Noodles, egg				
Cooked				
Dry	1 cup	213	2.4	53
Noodles, lasagna, cooked	2 oz.	216	2.4	54
Spaghetti	1 cup	197	0.9	0
Cooked				
Spaghetti twist, w/sauce, Buitoni	1 cup	155	0.6	0
	15 oz. can	300	8.0	0
POULTRY				
Chicken				
Breast, baked or broiled				
No skin				
With Skin	½ breast	142	3.0	82
Breast, fried, no skin, boneless	½ breast	193	7.6	79
With Skin	½ breast	161	4.1	75
Capon, w/skin, roasted	½ breast	338	17.0	111
Fryer, dark meat, no skin	3 oz.	195	9.9	73
Fried				
Roasted	3 oz.	203	9.9	82
Stewed	3 oz.	174	8.3	79
Fryer, dark meat w/skin	3 oz.	163	7.6	75
Floured, fried				
Roasted	3 oz.	242	14.2	78
Stewed	3 oz.	215	13.4	77
Fryer, white meat, no skin	3 oz.	198	12.5	70
Roasted				
Stewed	3 oz.	147	3.8	72
Fryer, white meat w/skin	3 oz.	135	3.4	65
Fried				
Roasted	3 oz.	163	4.7	77
Stewed	3 oz.	189	9.2	71
Fryer, heart, simmered	3 oz.	171	8.5	63
Fryer, wing meat, w/skin	3 oz.	157	6.7	206
Fried				
Roasted	3 oz.	276	18.5	67
Stewed	3 oz.	247	16.5	71
Giblets, cooked	1	100	6.7	28
Gizzards, simmered	3 oz.	1134	4.0	334
Leg, baked or broiled	3 oz.	130	3.1	165
No skin, drum/thigh				
With skin, drum/thigh				
Leg, fried, w/skin	1 each	178	7.8	87
Liver, cooked	1	260	15.1	103
Roaster, meat only roasted	1	431	25.5	142
	3 oz.	134	4.6	537
	3 oz.	142	5.6	64

CALORIES, FAT, AND CHOLESTEROL CONTENT OF SELECTED FOODS				
ITEM	**PORTION**	**CALORIES**	**FAT GRAMS**	**CHOLESTEROL mg**
POULTRY				
Stewing meat only, stewed				
No skin	3 oz.	202	10.1	71
With skin	3 oz.	242	16.0	67
Thigh cooked				
No skin	1	105	5.4	48
With skin	1	153	9.6	58
Poultry, Game				
Duck				
Domesticated, roasted	3 oz.	171	9.4	76
Pheasant, raw	3 oz.	113	3.1	-
Quail, raw	3 oz.	114	3.9	-
Goose, domesticated liver, raw	1	124	4.0	550
Roasted				
No skin	3 oz.	202	10.8	82
With skin	3 oz.	259	18.6	77
Turkey				
Light and dark, roasted, meat only				
No skin	3 oz.	145	4.2	65
With skin	3 oz.	177	8.3	70
Breast, w/skin	3 oz.	161	6.3	63
Dark meat, cooked				
No skin	3 oz.	159	6.1	72
With skin	3 oz.	188	9.8	76
RICE AND GRAINS				
Rice				
Brown, cooked	½ cup	108	0.9	0
Cakes, Chico San				
Buckwheat, no salt	1	36	0.2	0
With millet, no salt	1	36	0.2	0
Plain, no salt	1	36	0.2	0
Mix, chicken, Rice-A-Roni, Prepared	½ cup	107	0.7	-
White, cooked	½ cup	132	0.3	-
White, long grain				
Instant cooked	½ cup	81	0.1	0
Minute Rice	2/3 cup	120	0.0	0
Wild				
Uncooked	½ cup	286	0.9	0
Cooked	½ cup	83	0.3	0
Wild, long grain, Minute Rice, Cooked	½ cup	148	4.0	10

CALORIES, FAT, AND CHOLESTEROL CONTENT OF SELECTED FOODS				
ITEM	**PORTION**	**CALORIES**	**FAT GRAMS**	**CHOLESTEROL mg**
SALADS				
Beans, garbanzo, cooked, broiled and drained	2 tb.	3	0.0	0
Broccoli, raw, chopped	2 tb.	3	0.0	0
Carrots, raw, diced	2 tb.	7	0.0	0
Coleslaw, Regular, made w/mayonnaise	½ cup	41	1.6	5
Crouton	1	30	1.0	0
Cucumbers, raw, not pared	2 tb.	2	0.0	0
Lettuce	1 cup	7	0.1	0
Macaroni, made w/mayonnaise	½ cup	349	23.4	136
Mushrooms, raw	2 tb.	2	0.0	0
Onions, raw, chopped	2 tb.	8	0.0	0
Pasta w/seafood	1 cup	243	1.8	70
Peppers, green, raw, strips	½ cup	3	0.0	0
Tomatoes, fresh, chopped	1 tb.	5	0.0	0
SALAD DRESSINGS				
Blue Cheese, Kraft	1 tb.	76	7.6	4
Blue Cheese, low calorie				
Kraft	1 tb.	59	5.8	11
Wishbone	1 tb.	40	4.0	0
Blue Cheese, mix Good Season	1 tb.	3	0.0	0
Coleslaw, commercial	1 tb.	57	4.9	4
French				
Homemade	1 tb.	87	9.6	-
Kraft, Catalina	1 tb.	65	5.6	0
Kraft, regular	1 tb.	59	5.7	0
French, low-fat				
Kraft Free	1 tb.	20	0.0	0
Wishbone	1 tb.	2	0.0	0
Italian				
Bernstein's	1 tb.	32	1.0	0
Kraft, creamy	1 tb.	55	5.5	1
Kraft				
Italian, low-calorie				
Good Season, zesty, light	1 tb.	73	7.7	0

CALORIES, FAT, AND CHOLESTEROL CONTENT OF SELECTED FOODS				
ITEM	PORTION	CALORIES	FAT GRAMS	CHOLESTEROL mg
SALAD DRESSING				
Kraft	1 tb.	7	0.0	0
Wishbone	1 tb.	1	0.0	0
Italian, low-fat				
Kraft Free	1 tb.	6	0.0	0
No oil	1 tb.	8	0.0	0
Oil free, Kraft	1 tb.	4	0.0	0
Wishbone, creamy light	1 tb.	6	0.0	0
Mayonnaise				
Regular	1 tb.	99	10.9	8
Hellman's	1 tb.	98	10.8	10
Ranch, low-fat				
Kraft Free	1 tb.	16	0.0	0
Roka, reduced-calorie, Kraft	1 tb.	14	0.9	3
Russian	1 tb.	76	7.8	-
SNACKS				
Corn Chips				
Corn Snackers, Weight Watchers	1 oz.	121	4.0	-
Fritos	1 oz.	150	10.0	0
Black bean, garden	1 oz.	130	7.0	0
Doritos	1 oz.	140	6.0	0
Tostitos	1 oz.	140	8.0	0
Dips				
Avocado, Kraft	2 tb.	50	4.0	0
Blue cheese, Kraft, premium	2 tb.	45	4.0	10
Clam, Kraft	2 tb.	60	4.0	10
Guacamole	2 tb.	34	3.1	2
Onion, French, Kraft	2 tb.	60	4.0	0
Popcorn				
Air-popped	1 cup	23	0.3	0
Popped w/oil & salt	1 cup	41	2.0	0
Potato Chips				
Barbecue	1 oz.	152	9.4	0
Light, Pringles	1 oz.	130	6.0	0
Plain				
Cape Cod	1 oz.	150	8.0	0
Eagle	1 oz	150	10.0	0

CALORIES, FAT, AND CHOLESTEROL CONTENT OF SELECTED FOODS				
ITEM	**PORTION**	**CALORIES**	**FAT GRAMS**	**CHOLESTEROL mg**
Potato Chips				
Hawaiian	1 oz.	150	8.0	0
Pringles	1 oz.	160	11.0	0
Regular				
Lay's	1 oz.	150	10.0	0
Pringles	1 oz.	160	11.0	0
Ruffles	1 oz.	150	10.0	0
Pretzels				
Eagle	1 oz.	110	2.0	0
Mister Salty	1 oz.	109	1.1	0
Sticks, Mister Salty	10 sticks	101	0.0	0
No fat, thick, Snyder's	1 oz.	101	0.0	0
Soft commercial	1	145	0.4	0
Other Snacks				
Cheese Straws	1 oz.	128	8.4	-
Cheetos				
Crunchy	1 oz.	160	10.0	-
Light cheese snack	.9 oz.	120	6.0	-
Puffed balls	1 oz.	160	10.0	-
Corn nuts	1 oz.	129	4.3	0
Cracker Jacks	1 oz.	115	1.0	0
Fruit snacks, cherry,				
Grocer's choice	1 oz.	99	0.0	0
Fun Fruits, sunkist,	9 oz.	100	1.0	-
Funyuns	1 oz.	140	6.0	0
SOUPS				
Asparagus Cream of, canned				
Prepared w/water				
Prepared w/milk	1 cup	85	4.1	5
Beef bouillon	1 cup	161	7.9	22
Cubes dehydrated				
Granules, Herb-Ox	1	6	0.1	-
Beef consomme, canned	1 pkg.	8	0.0	-
w/water				
Beef Noodle	1 cup	31	0.0	24
Canned w/water				
Broth, chicken, low-fat	1 cup	83	3.1	5
Broth, chicken, Pritikin	1 cup	22	0.0	0
Chicken, cream of chicken	1 cup	16	0.0	0
And dumplings				
Chicken gumbo, Campbell	1 cup	96	5.5	34
Prepared	1 cup	55	1.2	-

CALORIES, FAT, AND CHOLESTEROL CONTENT OF SELECTED FOODS				
ITEM	**PORTION**	**CALORIES**	**FAT GRAMS**	**CHOLESTEROL mg**
SOUPS				
Chicken mushroom	1 cup	-	9.2	10
Chicken Noodles				
Dehydrated w/water	1 cup	53	1.2	3
Chicken Rice				
Dehydrated w/water	1 cup	61	1.4	3
Mix, w/gelatin, Corn	1 pkt.	78	0.1	0
chowder, homemade				
Lentil				
Homemade	1 cup	132	1.6	0
Minestrone				
Homemade	1 cup	113	1.7	2
Prepared, canned w/water	1 cup	82	2.5	2
Chunky, ready-to-serve	1 cup	127	2.8	5
Campbell	1 cup	92	2.4	-
Progresso	1 cup	30	1.8	2
Tabachnik	7.5 oz.	137	2.0	0
Dehydrated, prepared				
w/water	1 cup	79	1.7	3
Mushroom cream of, canned				
Prepared w/water				
Prepared w/milk	1 cup	129	9.0	2
With beef stock, prepared	1 cup	203	13.6	20
w/water				
Split pea, canned, *prepared,*	1 cup	85	4.0	7
w/water				
Tomato, canned				
Prepared w/milk	1 cup	190	4.3	8
Prepared w/water	1 cup	161	6.0	17
Tomato bisque, canned	1 cup	85	1.9	0
prepared w/water				
Tomato rice, canned,	1 cup	124	2.5	5
w/water				
Vegetable, vegetarian	1 cup	119	2.7	2
Campbell, prepared				
w/water				
Catsup				
Heinz	1 cup	78	1.2	0
Del Monte				
Heinz, low-salt	1 tb.	18	0.0	0
Olives	1 tb.	14	0.1	0
Black, ripe, pitted, medium	1 tb.	8	0.0	0
	2	9	0.9	0

CALORIES, FAT, AND CHOLESTEROL CONTENT OF SELECTED FOODS				
ITEM	**PORTION**	**CALORIES**	**FAT GRAMS**	**CHOLESTEROL mg**
SOUPS				
Pickle				
Sweet, whole	1 lg.	50	0.1	0
Pimento, canned				
Solids & liquid	2 tb.	9	0.1	0
Shake 'N' Bake				
Chicken, BBQ, dry	½ oz.	53	1.1	0
Soy sauce	1 tb.	8	0.0	0
Vinegar				
Cider	2 tb.	4	0.0	0
Distilled, white	2 tb.	4	0.0	0
VEGETABLES AND BEANS				
Baked, vegetarian				
Canned S&W	½ cup	115	1.0	0
Baked w/pork, canned				
Campbell	½ cup	120	1.5	9
Chickpeas, dried, boiled &				
Drained	½ cup	134	2.0	0
Kidney, dark red,				
Canned w/solids &				
Liquids	½ cup	109	0.0	0
Lentils, dried boiled and				
Drained	½ cup	115	0.0	0
Lima, baby, frozen				
Cooked, boiled and drained	½ cup	94	0.0	0
Lima, immature				
Dried, boiled and drained				
Lima, mature, dried,	½ cup	105	0.0	0
boiled and drained				
Mung, sprouted, seeds, raw	½ cup	108	0.0	0
Mung, sprouts, no seeds	½ cup	16	0.0	0
Pinto, cooked, boiled	½ cup	13	0.0	0
and drained				
Red, dried, boiled/drained	½ cup	117	0.0	0
Refried, canned, Old	½ cup	112	0.0	0
El Paso				
Refried, vegetarian	½ cup	130	2.0	-
Rosarita				
	½ cup	120	2.0	0

CALORIES, FAT, AND CHOLESTEROL CONTENT OF SELECTED FOODS				
ITEM	**PORTION**	**CALORIES**	**FAT GRAMS**	**CHOLESTEROL mg**
VEGETABLES AND BEANS				
Soybeans, cooked				
boiled & drained	½ cup	149	7.7	0
Split peas, cooked	½ cup	115	0.0	0
Sprouts	½ cup	16	0.0	0
Tempeh, fermented				
Soybean product	½ cup	165	6.4	0
Tofu, raw, firm	½ cup	183	11.0	0
White, small, cooked	½ cup	127	0.6	0
Vegetables & Potatoes				
Alfalfa sprouts	½ cup	5	0.0	0
Artichokes, fresh	1	53	0.2	0
Artichoke hearts, boiled,				
drained	½ cup	37	0.0	0
canned				
Asparagus	1 each	4	0.0	0
Canned, drained				
Beans, green, snap	½ cup	20	0.0	0
Frozen, cuts,	1	16	0.0	0
Beets, *fresh, cooked*				
Beets, red, pickled, canned	2 tb.	18	0.0	0
solids & liquid				
Beets, pickled, canned,	½ cup	74	0.0	0
solids & liquids				
Beet Greens (See Greens)	½ cup	12	0.0	0
Broccoli, fresh, *Raw*	5 oz.	110	5.0	-
Broccoli, frozen w/cheese	½ cup	30	0.0	0
sauce Birds Eye				
Brussel sprouts, fresh, cooked	½ cup	5	0.0	0
Cabbage, Chinese				
Cabbage, red				
Cooked	½ cup	16	0.0	0
Raw	½ cup	8	0.0	0
Cabbage, white				
Raw	½ cup	8	0.0	0
Carrots				
Raw				
Cauliflower, Cooked	1	31	0.0	0
Raw, florets	½ cup	15	0.0	0
Cauliflower, frozen, w/cheese	½ cup	19	0.0	0
sauce, Birds Eye				
	4 oz.	127	8.6	-

CALORIES, FAT, AND CHOLESTEROL CONTENT OF SELECTED FOODS				
ITEM	**PORTION**	**CALORIES**	**FAT GRAMS**	**CHOLESTEROL mg**
Vegetables & Potatoes				
Celery				
Cooked	½ cup	13	0.0	0
Fresh, stalk	1 each	6	0.0	0
Chinese, raw cabbage	½ cup	34	0.0	0
Collar greens (see Greens)				
Corn, sweet, fresh				
Yellow kernels	½ cup	90	0.0	0
White Kernels	½ cup	90	0.0	0
Corn, sweet, canned				
Cream style	½ cup	92	0.0	0
Corn on the cob	1 med.	80	0.0	0
Corn souffle	1 serv.	160	7.0	-
Cucumbers, whole, not pared	1	32	0.0	0
Eggplant, boiled and drained				
Endive, Belgian	½ cup	13	0.0	0
Escarole, raw	½ cup	7	0.0	0
Ginger root, raw	½ cup	4	0.0	0
Greens	½ cup	33	0.0	0
Collard, cooked and drained				
Mustard, boiled and drained	½ cup	12	0.0	0
Turnip				
Fresh, cooked	½ cup	10	0.0	0
Frozen, cooked				
Kale, cooked, leaves and				
stems	½ cup	14	0.0	0
Kohlrabi, thick, bulb only,	½ cup	25	0.0	0
cooked	½ cup	21	0.0	0
Leeks, bulb & lower leaf, cooked				
Lettuce, raw	½ cup	24	0.0	0
Butterhead	1 serv.	76	0.0	0
Crisphead, chopped				
Mixed, Italian, frozen				
Mushrooms	½ cup	4	0.0	0
Fresh, raw	½ cup	4	0.0	0
Canned, solids and liquids	½ cup	25	0.0	0
Okra, cooked	1	4	0.0	0
Onions	½ cup	15	0.0	0
Canned, french fried, Durkee	½ cup	26	0.0	0
Onion rings				
	½ cup	176	0.0	0
	1 oz.	276	0.0	0

CALORIES, FAT, AND CHOLESTEROL CONTENT OF SELECTED FOODS				
ITEM	PORTION	CALORIES	FAT GRAMS	CHOLESTEROL mg
Vegetables & Potatoes				
Parsley, fresh raw	½ cup	10	0.0	0
Parsnips, boiled and diced	½ cup	63	0.0	0
Peas & carrots, frozen, boiled and drained	½ cup	38	0.0	0
Peas, blackeye, cooked	½ cup	90	0.0	0
Peas, green, fresh cooked	½ cup	67	0.0	
Peas, green, canned Le Sueur, Green Giant	½ cup	102	4.4	0
Peas, snow, cooked	½ cup	34	0.0	0
Peppers				
Bell, chopped	½ cup	19	0.0	0
Hot chili				
Green, chopped	½ cup	30	0.0	0
Red, chopped	½ cup	29	0.0	0
Green, chopped	½ cup	19	0.0	0
Pimiento, canned solids & liquid	½ cup	35	0.0	0
Potatoes, Fresh				
Baked w/skin	1	218	0.0	0
Boiled	1	116	0.0	0
Boiled, pared, diced or sliced	½ cup	67	0.0	0
French-fried, homemade	½ cup	90	4.7	0
Potatoes, frozen				
French fried				
Cottage fries, Birds Eye	4 oz.	171	7.1	0
Birds Eye	1	37	1.3	0
Light, Ore-Ida	3 oz.	90	2.0	0
Hashbrown, shredded, Ore-Ida	½ cup	57	0.0	0
Boiled w/o skin, mashed	½ cup	172	0.0	0
Baked in skin	1	115	0.0	0
Yams, cooked, baked	½ cup	79	0.0	0
Rutabage, boiled sliced	½ cup	29	0.0	0
Scallions, raw	½ cup	16	0.0	0
Spinach, raw	½ cup	6	0.0	0
Squash				
Acorn				
boiled, mashed	½ cup	42	0.0	0

GLOSSARY

Glossary

I. Abbreviations, weights and measures

A. Abbreviations used

t	teaspoon
T	tablespoon
C	cup
oz	ounce

B. Common Household Measures

1T = 3t	1 pint = 2C
1C = 8 oz	2 pints = 1 quart
1C = 16 T	1 gallon = 2 quarts

C. Liquid Measures

1 litre = 1000 ml`	1t = 5 ml
1 C = 226.5 ml	1 pint = 20 oz.
1 T = 15 ml	

D. Weights

1 kg = 2.2 lbs.	1 lb. = 453.6 g
1 kg = 1000 g	1 lb. = 0.454 kg
1 oz. = 28.35 g	

II. Fahrenheit and Celsius Conversions for Oven Temperatures

A. Fahrenheit and Celsius Conversion

Fahrenheit	Celsius
300	150
350	180
375	190
400	200
435	220
450	230
475	240

B. Oven Temperatures

Warm	300 - 325^{0}F
Moderate	350 - 360^{0}F
Hot	375 - 400^{0}F
Very Hot	425 - 475^{0}F
Broiling	500^{0}F

III. Popular Indian (and South Asian) Foods

Baghar	Spices fried in oil and added to food. It is frequently used to garnish daals.
Bhara	Stuffed
Bharta	A cooked vegetable that is mashed.
Biryani	Rice and meat, or rice and vegetables cooked with various spices.
Chutney	Minced relish made from raw or sometimes cooked fruit or vegetables.
Daal	Curried lentils or pulses.
Garam masalla	Mixture of hot spices. See the recipe.
Ghee	Clarified butter
Keema	Minced meat.
Kheer	A sweet dessert made with cooking rice, lentils or tapioca or vermicelle, in milk.
Panir	Homemade cheese (see recipe on page 81).
Pullau	Curried rice dish.
Roita	Spiced yogurt with various types of grated or chopped fruits or vegetables.
Rati or Chappati	India bread.
Samosa	Deep fried triangular shaped snack, stuffed with minced meat or peas and potatoes.
Sivian	Thin vermicelli.

IV. Daals: Indian name for lentils

A. Nutritive Value: Daals are a very good source of protein and fiber.

B. Cooking Tips

1. Soak whole lentils overnight or soak in boiling water for ½ hour.
2. Split lentils can be soaked in cold water for 40 minutes before cooking.
3. Use the same water for cooking.
4. Add a couple of drops of oil during cooking to reduce foaming.
5. Do not use baking soda because it destroys the thiamin content of food.

C. Types of Daal (Commonly used Lentils)

1. Arhar daal - yellow-beige split lentil
2. Chana - similar to chick peas (garbanzo)
3. Chana daal - split golden pea lentil
4. Kala chana - small dark chick pea
5. Kali Mah - small black whole beans
6. Rajmah - red kidney beans
7. Masoor daal - orange-colored split lentil
8. Moong daal - yellow lentil hulled from the whole mung bean
9. Legumes with husk

    a. Moong - whole green mung beans
    b. Urad - small black beans, split

V. Commonly Used Spices

Asafetida (Heeng)	available as powder or in small lumps. Powdered asafetida is easier to use. It is added to hot oil followed by meats or vegetables
Bay leaf (Tez patta)	used as a garnish in Biryani and meat dishes
Cardamon (Elachi)	There are two kinds of cardamoms, large and small. Large ones are dark brown in color and are commonly used in meat preparation. Small cardamom is green in color and mostly used in tea and desserts.

Cinnamon (Dal Chini)	Cinnamon sticks are used in a variety of dishes. It can be also purchased in powdered form.
Clove (laung)	Laung is available in whole or powdered form. It is part of garam masalla.
Corriander (Dhania)	Green corriander is used as a garnish. Ground corriander is used in most Indian cooking.
Cumin (Zeera)	Available as seeds or powder. Roasted and then ground, the seeds add aroma to dishes.
Dill (Soya sag)	Used in some dishes.
Fennel (Saump)	Available as seed or powder. Powder is used in preparation of Kashmire style meats. Seeds are used as mints.
Fenugreek (methi)	Available as green leaves, dry powder or seeds.
Mustard (Sarson)	They are tiny, beadlike, reddish-brown to black color. They are used in pickles.
Nutmeg (Jaiphal)	Used in meat dishes and some desserts.
Onion Seeds (Kelonji)	Small black seeds, used in pickling.
Oregano Seeds (Ajwain)	Mostly used in bread and vegetable recipes.
Pomegranatt (Anar)	Dried and crushed seeds added to various dishes to give a tangy flavor.
Poppy seeds (Khas Khas)	Used in some curries.
Saffron (Zahaan)	Extracted from Saffron flowers and used to give aroma and a golden yellow color. Saffron is frequently used in pillau's and some meat dishes.
Tamarind (Imli)	Known for its sweet-fourtell pulp diluted with water, tamarind used to give a tangy taste to the food.
Tumeric (Haldi)	Available in dried and powdered form. It is yellow in color.

VI. Heart-Diet Terminology

Atherosclerosis — A condition caused by the build up of fatty material and other substances that clog and reduce the elasticity of the inner layer of the arterial wall. As this condition progresses, the openings of the arteries gradually close up and the blood supply is reduced.

Bile — Fluid secreted by the liver; an important aid to digestion and fat absorption.

Calorie — Unit of measurement used to give a numerical expression to the amount of energy in food.

Carbohydrate — One of the three nutrients that supply energy to the body. Carbohydrates provide four calories per gram. There are two kinds of carbohydrates, simple and complex.

- Simple carbohydrates (sugars) are found in cookies, cakes and pies, Indian sweets (Mithai) and other man-made and natural foods.

- Complex carbohydrates originate in plants and are found in starch and fiber. Foods high in **starch** include breads, cereals, pasta, rice, dried beans, peas, and corn. **Fiber** is nondigestible and is found in whole grain breads and cereals, whole fruits and dried beans. It comes in two forms, soluble and insoluble; soluble fiber is found in oat and barley bran, apples and oranges, and some dried beans, and may be helpful in reducing blood cholesterol.

Cholesterol — a soft, waxy substance occurring naturally throughout the body, including the blood, and important to the production of cells and hormones. Cholesterol is produced by the liver and other organs. Major food sources of cholesterol are egg yolks, meat, organ meats and dairy products. High levels of blood cholesterol increase the risk of heart disease.

Fat — One of the three nutrients that supply calories to the body. One gram of fat provides nine calories. Fat takes two major forms: saturated and unsaturated;

- Major sources of **saturated fats** are animal fats and whole milk dairy products. Vegetable oils such as coconut and palm oils are particularly high in saturated fat content. Saturated fat raises blood cholesterol.

- **Unsaturated fats** are generally in a liquid state at refrigerator temperatures. They are divided into two types: **monounsaturated** and **polyunsaturated fat**. **Monounsaturated** fat is found in olive and rapeseed (canola) oil. **Polyunsaturated** fat is derived mainly from plants, including safflower, corn and soybean oil. Both **monounsaturated** and **polyunsaturated** fats help reduce blood cholesterol, and should be used in place of **saturated** fats. {Note: You can calculate the percentage of calories from fat by using the following equation:

$$\frac{\text{Grams of Fat} \times 9}{\text{Total Calories}} \times 100$$

Example: 2 slices of pizza has 400 calories and 8 grams of fat, thus the percentage of calories from fat would be shown as $\frac{8 \times 9}{400} \times 100 = 18$.

Hydrogenation — A chemical process that transforms liquid vegetable oils (unsaturated fat) into denser saturated fat.

Lipids — Fatty substances, including cholesterol and triglycerides, present in blood and body tissue.

Lipoprotein — Protein-coated substances that carry fat and cholesterol through the blood. Lipoprotein is classified according to **high** and **low** density;

- **High density lipoprotein (HDL)** contains a small amount of cholesterol and transports it out of the body's cells to the liver where it is processed for disposal. Low levels of HDL are associated with an increased risk of coronary heart disease.

- **Low density lipoprotein (LDL)** contains the largest amount of cholesterol in the blood. LDL is responsible for depositing cholesterol in the arterial walls. Thus, high levels of LDL are associated with an increased risk of coronary heart disease. {Note: If the ratio of total cholesterol to HDL cholesterol exceeds 5.0, or the ratio of LDL cholesterol to HDL cholesterol exceeds 4.0, there is a high risk of developing coronary heart disease.}

Protein	One of the three nutrients that supply calories to the body. One gram of protein provides four calories.
Triglycerides	A fat containing one glycerol (alcohol) and three fatty acids. Most body fat is stored in triglyceride form. The primary source of triglycerides is from the fat consumed in one's diet.

REFERENCES

1. Abate, N, Garg, A, Enas, EA. Physico-chemical properties of low-density lipoproteins in normo-lipidemic Asian Indian men. Horm Metab Res. 1995;27:326-331.

2. Abdel-Maksoud, MD, Hokanson, JE. The complex role of triglycerides in cardiovascular disease. Semin Vasc Med. 2002;2:325-333.

3. American Diabetes Association. Nutrition principles and recommendations in diabetes. Diabetes Care. 2004;27(suppl):S36-S46.120.

4. American Dietetic Association. Indian and Pakistani Food Practices, Customs, and Holidays. 2nd ed. Ethnic and Regional Food Practices series. Chicago, Ill: American Dietetic Association; 2000.

5. American Heart Association, Heart Attack, Treatment, Recovery, Prevention. American Heart Association, Inc., 1996.

6. Anderson, J. Dietary fiber prevents carbohydrate-induced hypertriglyceridemia. Curr Athero Rep. 2000;2:536-541.

7. Anderson, KM, Castelli, WP, Levy, D. Cholesterol and mortality: 30 years of follow-up from the Framingham Study. JAMA. 1987;257:2176-2180.

8. Angelin, B. Therapy for lowering lipoprotein(a) levels. Curr Opin Lipidol. 1997;8:337-341.

9. Anand, SS, Yusuf, S, Vuksan, V, et al. Differences in risk factors, atherosclerosis, and cardiovascular disease between ethnic groups in Canada: The Study of Health Assessment and Risk in Ethnic groups (SHARE). Lancet, 2000;356:279-284.

10. Anand, SS, Enas, EA, Pogue, J, Haffner, S, Pearson, T, Yusuf, S. Elevated lipoprotein(a) levels in South Asians in North America. Metabolism. 1998;47(2):182-184.

11. Assmann, G, Schulte, H, Funke, H, von Eckardstein, A. The emergence of triglycerides as a significant independent risk factor in coronary artery disease. Eur Heart J. 1998;19(suppl M):M8-M14.

12. Austin, MA, Breslow, JL, Hennekens, CH, Buring, JE, Willett, WC, Krauss, RM. Low-density lipoprotein subclass patterns and risk of myocardial infarction. JAMA. 1988;260:1917-1921.

13. Austin, MA, King, M-C, Vranizan, KM, Krauss, RM. Atherogenic lipoprotein phenotype: a proposed genetic marker for coronary heart disease risk. Circulation. 1990;82:495-506.

14. Ballantyne, CM, Herd, JA, Ferlic, LL, Dunn, JK Farmer, JA, Jones, PH, Schein, JR, Gotto, AM Jr. Influence of low HDL on progression of coronary artery disease and response to fluvastatin therapy. Circulation. 1999;99:736-743.

15. Banerji, MA, Faridi, N, Athluri, R, Chaiken, RL, Lebovitz, HE. Body composition, visceral fat, leptin, and insulin resistance in Asian Indian men. J Clin Endocrinol Metab. 1999;84:137-144.

16. Barter, PJ, Rye, KA. High density lipoproteins and coronary heart disease. Atherosclerosis. 1996;121:1-12.

17. *Basic Food Preparation, a Complete Manual.* Orient Longman Limited, New Delhi, India, 1986.

18. Baylin, A, Kabagambe, EK, Ascherio, A, Spiegelman, D, Campos, H. High 18:2 trans fatty acids in adipose tissue are associated with increased risk of nonfatal acute myocardial infarction in Costa Rican adults. J Nutr. 2003; 133:1186-1191.

19. Bhalodkar, NC, Blum, S, Rana, T, et al. Comparison of levels of large and small high-density lipoprotein cholesterol in Asian Indian men compared with Caucasian men in the Framingham Offspring Study. Am J Cardiol. 2004;94(12):1561-1563.

20. Becker, DM, Becker, LC, Pearson, TA, Fintel, DJ, Levine, DM, Kwiterovich, PO. Risk factors in siblings of people with premature coronary heart disease. J Am Coll Cardiol. 1988;12:1273-1280.

21. Bhalodkar, NC, Blum, S, Rana, T, Kitrchappa, R, Bhalodkar, AN, Enas, RA. Comparison of high-density and low-density lipoprotein cholesterol subclasses and sizes in Asian Indian women with caucasian women from the Framingham Offspring Study. Clin Cardiol. 2005;28(5):247-251.

22. Bhatnagar, D, Anan, IS, Durrington, PN, Patel, DJ, Wander, GS, Mackness, NI, Creed, F. Tomenson, B, Chandrashekhar, Y, Winterbotham, M, Britt, RP, Keil, JE, Sutton, GC. Coronary risk factors in people from the Indian subcontinent living in West London and their siblings in India. Lancet. 1995;345:405-409.

23. Bierman, EL. George Lyman Duff Memorial Lecture. Atherogenesis in diabetes. Arterioscler Throm. 1992;12:647-656.

24. Bray, GA, Champagne, CM. Obesity and the metabolic syndrome: implications for dietetics practitioners. J Am Diet Assoc. 2003;104:86-89.

25. Budde, T, Fechtrup, C, Bosenber, E, Vielhauer C, Enbergs, A. Schulte, H, Assmann, G, Breithardt, G. Plasma Lp(a) levels correlate with number, severity, and lenght-extension of coronary lesions in male patient undergoing coronary arteriography for clinically suspected coronary atherosclerosis. Arteioscler Thromb. 1994;14:1730-1736.

26. Chambers, JC, Kooner, JS. Homocysteine: a novel risk factor for coronary heart disease in UK Indian Asians. Heart. 2001;86:121-122.

27. Chandalia, M, Garg, A, Luthjohann, D, von Bergmann, K, Grundy, SM, Brinkley, LJ. Beneficial effects of high dietary fiber intake in patients with type 2 diabetes mellitus. N Engl J Med. 2000;342:1392-1398.

28. Corti, M-C, Guralnik, JM, Salive, ME, Harris, T, Field, TS, Wallace, RB, Berkman, LF, Seeman, TE, Glynn, RJ, Hennekens, CH, Havlik, RJ. HDL cholesterol predicts coronary heart disease mortality in older persons. JAMA. 1995;274:539-544.

29. Criqui, MH, Langer, RD, Fronek, A, Feigelson, HS, Klauber, MR, McCann, TJ, Browner, D. Mortality over a period of 10 years in patients with peripheral arterial disease. N Engl J Med. 1992;236:381-386.

30. Danesh, J, Collins, R, Peto, R. Lipoprotein(a) and coronary heart disease: meta-analysis of prospective studies. Circulation. 2000;102:1082-1085.

31. Das, UN, Kumar, KV, Ramesh, G. Essential fatty acid metabolism in South Indians. Prostglandins Leukot Essent Fatty Acids. 1994;50:253-255.

32. de Lorgeril, M. Salen, P, Martin, JL, Monjaud, I, Delaye, J, Mamell, N. Mediterranean diet, traditional risk factors, and the rate of cardiovascular complications after myocardial infarction: final report of the Lyon Diet Heart Study. Circulation. 1999;99:779-785.

33. Dengel, DR, Galecki, AT, Hagberg, JM, Pratley, RE. The independent and combined effects of weight loss and aerobic exercise on blood pressure and oral glucose tolerance in older men. Am J Hypertens. 1998;11:1405-1412.

34. Denke, MA, Sempos, CT, Grundy, SM. Excess body weight: an underrecognized contributor to high blood cholesterol levels in white American men. Arch Intern Med. 1993;153:1093-1103.

35. Denke, MA, Adams-Huet, B, Nguyen, AT. Individual cholesterol variation in response to a margarine- or butter-based diet: a study in families. JAMA. 2000;284:2740-2747.

36. Deurenberg, P, Deurenberg-Yap, M, Guricci, S. Asians are different from Caucasians and from each other in their body mass index/body fat per cent relationship. Obes Rev. 2002;3:141-146.

37. Deurenberg-Yap, M, Chew, SK, Deurenberg, P. Elevated body fat percentage and cardiovascular risks at low body mass index levels among Singaporean Chinese, Malays and Indians. Obes Rev. 2002;3:209-215.

38. Diabetes Prevention Program Research Group. Reduction in the incidence of type 2 diabetes with lifestyle intervention or metformin. N Engl J Med. 2002;346:393-403.

39. Dolecek, TA, Stamler, J, Caggiula, A, Tillotson, JL, Buzzard, IM. Methods of dietary and nutritional assessment and intervention and other methods in the Multiple Risk Factor Intervention Trial. Am J Clin Nutr. 1997;65(suppl):196S-210S.

40. Dris-Etherton, PM, Etherton, TD, Carlson, J, Gardner, C. Recent discoveries in inclusive food-based approaches and dietary patterns for reduction in risk for cardiovascular disease. Curr Opin Lipidol. 2002;12:397-407.

41. Dudeja, V, Misra, A, Pandey, RM, Devina, G, Kumar, G, Vikram, NK. BMI does not accurately predict overweight in Asian Indians in northern India. Br J Nutr. 2001;86:105-112.

42. Eating To Lower Your Blood Cholesterol, U.S. Department of Health and Human Services, Public Health Service, National Institutes of Health, 1989.

43. Eckel, RH, Krauss, RM, for the AHA Nutrition Committee. American Heart Association call to action: obesity as a major risk factor for coronary heart disease. Circulation. 1998;97:2099-2100.

44. Eikelboom, JW, Lonn E, Genst, J Jr, Hankey G, Uusuf S. Homocysteine and cardiovascular disease: a critical review of the epidemiologic evidence. Ann Intern Med. 1999;131:363-375.

45. Elias, SL, Innis, SM. Bakery foods are the major dietary source of trans-fatty acids among pregnant women with diets providing 30 percent energy from fat. J Am Diet Assoc. 2002;102:46-51.

46. Enas, EA, Mehta, J. Malignant coronary artery disease in young Asian Indians: thoughts on pathogenesis, prevention, and therapy. Clin Cardiol. 1995;18:131-135.

47. Enas, EA. Rapid angiographic progression of coronary artery disease in patients with elevated lipoprotein(s). Circulation. 1995;92:2353-2354.

48. Enas, EA, Davidson, MA, Garg, A, Nair, VM, Yusuf, S. Prevalence of coronary heart disease and its risk factors in Asian Indian migrants to the US. Indian Heart J. 1996;48(4):343-353.

49. Enas, Enas A: Prevention of Heart Attacks in Indians. *Journal of American Association of Indian Physicians*. 6 (1), 25-26, 1994.

50. Enas, EA. Coronary artery disease epidemic in Indians: A cause for alarm and call for action. J Indian Med Assoc. 2000;98(11):694-695, 697-702.

51. Enas, EA. Clinical implications: Dyslipidemia in the Asian Indian Population. Oakbrook Terrace, Ill: 2002. American Association of Physicians of Indian Origin.

52. Enas, EA, Senthilkumar, A, Juturu, V, Gupta, R. Coronary artery disease in women. Indian Heart J. 2001;53(3):282-292.

53. Enas, EA, Garg, A, Davidson, MA, Nair, YM, Huet, BA, Yusuf, S. Coronary heart disease and its risk factors in first-generation immigrant Asian Indians to the United States of America. Indian Heart J. 1996;48(4):343-353.

54. Enas, EA, Mehtra, J. Malignant coronary artery disease in young Asian Indians: Thoughts on pathogenesis, prevention, and therapy. Coronary Artery Disease in Asian Indians (CADI) Study. Clin Cardiol. 1995;18(3):131-135.

55. Enas, EA, Senthikumar, A, Vinod, C, Puthumana, N. Dyslipideaemia among Indo-Asians: Strategies for identification and management. Br J Diabetes Vasc Dis. 2005;5(2):81-90.

56. Expert Committee on the Diagnosis and Classification of Diabetes Mellitus, The. Follow-up report on the diagnosis of diabetes mellitus. Diabetes Care. 2003;26:3160-3176.

57. Expert Panel on Detection, Evaluation, and Treatment of High Blood Cholesterol in Adults. Executive summary of the third report of the National Cholesterol Education (NCEP) Expert Panel on Detection, Evaluation, and Treatment of High Blood Cholesterol in Adults (Adult Treatment Panel III). JAMA. 2001;285(19):2486-2497.

58. Expert Panel on Detection, Evaluation, and Treatment of High Blood Cholesterol in Adults. Executive summary of the Third Report of the National Cholesterol Education Program (NCEP) Expert Panel on Detection, Evaluation, and Treatment of High Blood Cholesterol in Adults (Adult Treatment Panel III). JAMA 2001;285:2485-2497. Full report: National Institutes of Health. Third Report of the National Cholesterol Education Program Expert Panel on Detection, Evaluation, and Tretment of High Blood Cholesterol in Adults (Adult Treatment Panel III). Bethesda, Md: National Institutes of Health; 2001. NIH Publication 01-3670. Available at: http://www.nhlbi.nih.gov/guidelines/cholesterol/atp3_rpt.htm. Accessed March 29, 2004.

59. Farrell, SW, Kampert, JB, Kohl, HW III, Barlow, CE, Macera, CA, Paffenbarger, RS Jr, Gibbons, LW, Blair, SN. Influences of cardiorespiratory fitness levels and other predictors on cardiovascular disease mortality in men. Med Sci Sports Exerc. 1998;30:899-905.

60. Flegal, KM, Carroll, MD, Ogden, CL, Johnson, CL. Prevalence and trends in obesity among US adults, 1999-2000. JAMA. 2002;288:1723-1727.

61. Ford, E. Giles, W, Dietz, W. Prevalence of the metabolic syndrome among US adults. JAMA. 2002;287:356-359.

62. Ford, ES, Giles, WH. A comparison of the prevalence of the metabolic syndrome using two proposed definitions. Diabetes Care. 2003;26:575-581.

63. Frank, S.J. and Stone, K. *Fat, Sodium, Cholesterol and Calorie Counter.* Globe Communications, Corporation, 1996.

64. Garg, A. High-monounsaturated-fat diets for patients with diabetes mellitus: a meta-analysis. Am J Clin Nutr. 1998;67(suppl):577S-582S.

65. Gestein, HC, Pais, P, Pogue, J, Yusuf, S. Relationship of glucose and insulin levels to the risk of myocardial infarction: a case-control study. J Am Coll Cardiol. 1999;33:612-619.

66. Ginsberg, HN. New perspectives on atherogenesis. Role of abnormal triglyceride-rich lipoprotein metabolism. Circulation. 2002;106:2137-2142.

67. Grundy, SM. Comparison of monounsaturated fatty acids and carbohydrates for lowering plasma cholesterol. N Engl J Med. 1986;314:745-748.

68. Grundy, SM. Nutrition and diet in the management of hyperlipidemia and atherosclerosis. In: Shils, ME, Olson, JA, Shike, M, Ross, AC, eds. Modern Nutrition in Health and Disease. 9th ed. Baltimore, Md: Williams & Wilkins; 1999:1199-1216.

69. Grundy, SM. What is the desirable ratio of saturated, polyunsaturated, and monunsaturated fatty acids in the diet? Am J Clin Nutr. 1997;66(suppl):988S-990S.

70. Gupta, R, Kastia, S, Kaul, V, Nagar, R, Enas, EA. Lipoprotein(a) in coronary artery disease: A case-control study. Indian Heart J. 2000;52(4):407-410.

71. Haffner, SM. Impaired glucose tolerance: is it relevant for cardiovascular disease? Diabetologia. 1997;40(suppl):S138-S140.

72. Hansen, EF, Anderson, LT, Von Eyben, FE. Cigarette smoking and age at first acute myocardial infarction, and influence of gender and extent of smoking. Am J Cardiol. 1993;71:1439-1442.

73. Harnack, L, Lee, S, Schakel, SF, Duval, S, Luepker, RV, Arnett, DK. Trends in the trans-fatty acid composition of the diet in a metropolitan area: The Minnesota Heart Survey. J Am Diet Assoc. 2003;103:1160-1166.

74. Hartz, AJ, Rupley, DC, Kalkhoff, RD, Rimm, AA. Relationship of obesity to diabetes: influence of obesity level and body fat distribution. Prev Med. 1983:12:351-357.

75. Heart Protection Study Collaborative Group. MRC/BHF Heart protection Study of cholesterol-lowering with simvastatin in 5963 people with diabetes: a randomized placebo-controlled trial. Lancet. 2003;361:2005-2016.

76. Helmrich, SP, Ragland, Dr, Leung, RW, Paffenbarger, RS Jr. Physical activity and reduced occurrence of noninsulin-dependent diabetes mellitus. N Engl J Med. 1991;325:147-152.

77. Hjermann, I, Holme, I, Velve, BK, Leren, P. Effect of diet and smoking intervention on the incidence of coronary heart disease: report from the Oslo Study Group of a randomized trial in healthy men. Lancet. 1981;2:1303-1310.

78. Hoogeveen, RC, Gambhir, JK, Gambhir, DS, et al. Evaluation of Lp(a) and other independent risk factors for CHD in Asian Indians and their USA counterparts. J Lipid Res. 2001;42:631-638.

79. Hu, FB, Stampfer, MJ, Solomon, C, Liu, S, Colditz, GA, Speizer, FE, Willett, WC, Manson, JE. Physical activity and risk for cardiovascular events in diabetic women. Ann Intern Med. 2001;134:96-105.

80. Institute of Medicine. Dietary Reference Intakes: Energy, Carbohydrate, Fiber, Fat, Fatty Acids, Cholesterol, Protein, and Amino Acids. Washington, DC: National Academies Press, 2002.

81. Isomaa, B, Henricsson, M, Almgren, P, Tuomi, T, Taskinen, MR, Groop, L. The metabolic syndrome influences the risk of chronic complications in patients with type II diabetes. Diabetologia. 2001;44:1148-1154.

82. Jacques, PF, Bostom, AG, Williams, RR, Ellison, RC, Eckfeldt, JH, Rosenberg, IH, Sellub, J. Rozen, R. Relation between folate status, a common mutation in methylenetetrahydrofolate reductase, and plasma homocysteine concentrations. Circulation. 1996;93:7-9.

83. Jacques, PF, Selhub, J. Boston, AG, Wilson, PWF, Rosenberg, IH. The effect of folic acid fortification on plasma folate and total homocysteine concentrations. N Engl J Med. 1999;340:1449-1454.

84. Judd, J, Baer D, Clevidence B, Kris-Etherton, P, Musesing, R. Dietary cis and trans monounsaturated and saturated fatty acids. Lipids. 2002;37:123-131.

85. Kamath, SK, Ravishanker, C, Briones, E, Chen, EH. Macronutrient intake and blood cholesterol level of a community of Asian Indians living in the United States. J Am Diet Assoc. 1997;97:299-301.

86. Kang, SS, Wong, PWK, Malinow, MR. Hyperhomocyst(e)inemia as a risk factor for occlusive vascular disease. Ann Rev Nutr. 1992;12:279-298.

87. Kaul, Lalita; Brown, Melani; Wilson, Marcia; Ulep, Diosdado; Nidiry, Joseph: High Fiber Diet in the Treatment of Obesity. *International Clinical Review.* 7 (4), 174-179, 1987.

88. Kaul, L, Nidiry, JJ, Williams, HW. Multidisciplinary approach to the management of obesity. Medical and Engineering Publishers Inc.; Maryland 2005.

89. Klein, R. Kelly West Lecture 1994: hyperglycemia and microvascular and macrovascular disease in diabetes. Diabetes Care. 1995;18:258-268.

90. Klem, ML, Wing, RR, McGuire, MT, Seagle, HM, Hill, JO. A descriptive study of individuals successful at long-term maintenance of substantial weight loss. Am J Clin Nutr. 1998;66:239-249.

91. Knight, TM, Smith, Z, Whittles A, Sahota, P, Hogg, G, Bedford, A. Insulin resistance, diabetes, and risk markers for ischemic heart disease in Asian men and non-Asian men in Bradfor. Br Heart J. 1992;67:343-350.

92. Koba, S, Hirano, T, Kondo, T, Shibata, M, Suzuki, H, Murakami, M, Geshi, E, Katagiri, T. Significance of small dense low-density lilpoproteins and other risk factors in patients with various types of coronary heart disease. Am Heart J. 2002;144:1026-2035.

93. Krauss, RM, Dreon, DM. Low-density-lipoprotein subclasses and response to a low-fat in healthy men. Am J Clin Nutr. 1995;62(suppl):478S-487S.

94. Kris-Etherton, PM, Pearson, TA, Wan, Y, Hargrove, RL, Moriarty, K, Fishell, V, Etherton, TD. High-monounsaturated fatty acid diets lower both plasma cholesterol and triacylglycerol concentrations. Am J Clin Nutr. 1999;70:1009-1015.

95. Kris-Etherton, PM. Monounsaturated fatty acids and risk of cardiovascular disease. Circulation. 1999;100:1253-1258.

96. Krieger, DR, Landsberg, L. Mechanisms in obesity-related hypertension: role of insulin and catecholamines. Am J Hypertens. 1998;1:84-90.

97. Kulkami, KR, Markovitz, JH, Nanda, NC, Segrest, JP. Increased prevalence of smaller and denser LDL particles in Asian Indian. Arterioscler Thromb Vasc Biol. 1999;19:2749-2755.

98. Kulkami, KR, Markovitz, JH, Nanda, NC, Segrest, JP. Increased prevalence of smaller and denser LDL particles in Asian Indians. Arterioscler Thromb Vasc Biol. 1999;19:2749-2755.

99. Kuppuswamy, V, Gupta, S. Coronary heart disease in South Asians. Practitioners. 2003;247:181-182,186-188.

100. Kwiterovich, P. *The Johns Hopkins Complete Guide for Avoiding Heart Disease -- Beyond Cholesterol.* The Johns Hopkins University Press. Baltimore and London, 1989.

101. Lada, AT, Rudel, LL. Dietary monounsaturated versus polyunsaturated fatty acids: which is really better for protection from coronary heart disease? Curr Opin Lipidol. 2003;12:41-46.

102. Laws, A, Jeppesan, JL, Maheusx, PC, Schaaf, Chen, YD, Reaven, GM. Resistance to insulin-stimulated glucose uptake and dyslipidemia in Asian Indians. Arterioscler Thromb. 1994;14:917-922.

103. Lichtenstein, AH, Erkkila, AT, Lamarche, B, Schwab, US, Jalbert, SM, Ausman, LM. Influence of hydrogenated fat and butter on CVD risk factors remnant like particles, glucose and insulin, blood pressure and C-reactive protein. Atherosclerosis. 2003;171:97-107.

104. Liem, A, Reynierse-Buitenwerf GH, Zwinderman, AH, Jukema JW, van Veldhuisen DJ. Secondary prevention with folic acid: effects on clinical outcomes. J Am Coll Cardiol. 203;41:2105-2113.

105. Liew, CF, Seah, ES, Yeo, KP, Lee, KO, Wise, SD. Lean, nondiabetic Asian Indians have decreased insulin sensitivity and insulin clearance, and raised leptin compared with Caucasians and Chinese subjects. Int J Obes Relat Metab Disord. 2003;27:784-789.

106. McKeigue, PM, Shah, B, Marmot, MG. Relation of central obesity and insulin resistance with high diabetes prevalence and cardiovascular risk in South Asians. Lancet. 1991;337:382-386.

107. Maher, VM, Brown, BG, Marcovina, SM, Hillger, LA, Zhao, XQ, Albers, JJ. Effects of lowering elevated LDL cholesterol on the cardiovascular risk of lipoprotein(s). JAMA. 1995;274:1771-1774.

108. Manolio, TA, Pearson, TA, Wenger, NK, Barrett-Connor, E, Payne, GH, Harlan, WR. Cholesterol and heart disease in older persons and women: review of an NHLBI workshop. Ann Epidemiol. 1992;2:161-176.

109. Mauger, J-F, Lichenstein, AH, Ausman, LM, Jalber, SM, Jauhiainen, M, Ehnholm, C, Lamarche, B. Effect of different forms of dietary hydrogenated fats on LDL particle size. Am J Clin Nutr. 2003;78:370-375.

110. Mehta, Shahnaze and Korenblit, Joan. *Good Cooking from India*. Rodale Press, Emmaus, Pennsylvania, 1981.

111. Meigs, JB. Invited commentary: insulin resistance syndrome? Syndrome X? Multiple metabolic syndrome? A syndrome at all? Factor analysis reveals patterns in the fabric of correlated metabolic risk factors. Am J Epidemiol. 2000;152:908-911.

112. Mensink, RP, Sock, PL, Kester, ADM, Katan, MB. Effects of dietary fatty acids and carbohydrates on the ratio of serum total to HDL cholesterol and on serum lipids and apolipoproteins: a meta-analysis of 60 controlled trials. Am J Clin Nutr. 2003;77:1146-1155.

113. Miller, GJ, Kotecha, S, Wilkinson, WH, Wilkes, H, StirlingY, Sanders, TA, Broad, A, Allison, J, Meade, TW. Dietary and other characteristics relevant for coronary heart disease in man of Indian, West Indian and European descent in Longon. Atherosclerosis. 1988;70:63-72.

114. Mirkin, Gabe. *Fat Counter*. Linx Corporation, P.O. Box 613, Great Falls, Virginia 22066, 1995.

115. Mohan, V, Deppa, R, Rani, SS, Premalatha,, G. Prevalence of coronary artery disease and its relationship to lipids in a selected population in South India: The Chenna Urban Population Study (CUPS No. 5). J Am Coll Cardiol. 2001;38(3):682-687.

116. Moliterno, DJ, Jokinen, EV, Miserez, AR, Lange, RA, Willard, JE, Boerwinkle, E, Hilis, LD, Hobbs, HH. No association between plasma lipoprotein(a) concentrations and the presence or absence of coronary atherosclerosis in African Americans. Arterioscler Thomb Vasc Biol. 1995;15:850-855.

117. National Heart, Lung, and Blood Institute Third Report of the National Cholesterol Education Program Expert Panel on Detection, Evaluation, and Treatment of High Blood Cholesterol in Adults (Adult Treatment Panel III). Executive Summary. Bethesda, Md: National Institutes of Health; 2001. NIH publication 01-3670.

118. National Institutes of Health. Clinical guidelines on the identification, evaluation, and treatment of overweight and obesity in adults – the evidence report. Bethesda, Md: National Heart, Lung and Blood Institute; 1998. NIH publication 98-4083. Available at: www.nhlbi.nih.gov/guidelines/obesity/ob_home.htm. Accessed March 29, 2004.

119. National Institutes of Health/National Heart, Lung, and Blood Institute/Obesity Education Initiative Expert Panel. Clinical Guidelines on the Identification, Evaluation, and Treatment of Overweight and Obesity in Adults. The Evidence Report. NIH; 1998. Available at http://www.nhlbi, nih.gov/about/oei/index.htm. Accessed December 10, 2003.

120. Ness, AR, Powles, JW. Fruits and vegetables and cardiovascular disease: a review. Int J Epoidemiol. 1997;26:1-13.

121. Nishino, M, Malloy, MJ, Naya-Vigne, J, Russell, J, Kane, JP, Redberg, RF. Lack of association of lipoprotein(a) levels with coronary calcium deposits in asymptomatic postmenopausal women. J Am Coll Cardiol. 2000;35:314-320.

122. Nyboe, J, Jensen, G, Appelyard, M, Schnohr, P. Smoking and the risk of first acute myocardial infarction. Am Heart J. 1991;122:438-447.

123. Okosun, IS, Choi, ST, Boltri, JM, Parish, DC, Chandra, KM, Dever, GE, Lucas, A. Trends of abdominal adiposity in white, black, and Mexican-American adults, 1988 to 2000. Obes Res. 2003;11:1010-1017.

124. Okosun, IS, Liao, Y, Rotimi, CN, Prewitt, TE, Cooper, RS. Abdominal adiposity and clustering of multiple metabolic syndrome in white, black and Hispanic Americans. Ann Epidemiol. 2000;10:263-270.

125. Ornish, D, Scherwitz, LW, Billings, JH, Brown, SF, Gould KI, Merritt, TA, Sparler, S, Armstrong, WT, Ports, TA, Kirkeeide, RL, Hogeboom, D, Brand, RJ. Intensive lifestyle changes for reversal of coronary heart disease. JAMA. 1998;280:2001-2007.

126. Ornish, Dean. *Eat More, Weigh Less*. Harper Collins, 1993.

127. Paffenbarger, RS Jr, Hyde, RT, Wing, AL, Lee I-M, Jung DL, Kampert, JB. The association of changes in physical-activity level and other lifestyle characteristics with mortality among men. N Engl J Med. 1993;328:538-545.

128. Park, Y, Zhu, S, Palaniappan, L, Heshka, S, Carnethon, MR, Heymsfield, SB. The metabolic syndrom: prevalence and associated risk factors findings in the US population from the Third National Health and Nutrition Examination Survey, 1988-1994. Arch Intern Med. 2003;163:427-436.

129. Palaniappan, L, Wang, Y, Fortmann, SP. Coronary heart disease mortality for six ethnic groups in California. 1990-2000. Ann Epidemiol. 2004;14(7):499-506.

130. Pohjola-Sintonen, S, Rissanen, A, Liskola, P, Luomanmaki, K. Family history as a risk factor of coronary heart disease in patients under 60 years of age. Eur Heart J. 1998;19:235-239.

131. Pope-Cordle, J and Kaahn, Martin. *The T-factor, Fat Gram Counter.* W.W. Norton & Company, New York, London, 1994.

132. Raji, A, Seely, EW, Arky,RA, Simonson, DC. Body fat distribution and insulin resistance in health Asian Indians and Caucasians. J Clin Endocrinol Metab. 2001;86:5366-5371.

133. Roth, Harriet. *Fat Counter.* Penguin Books, U.S.A., Inc., New York, 1992.

134. Rissanen, AM, Nikkila, E. Coronary artery disease and its risk factors in families of young men with angina pectoris and in controls. Br Heart J. 1977;39:875-883.

135. Sacks, FM, Campos, H. Low-density lipoprotein size and cardiovascular disease: a reappraisal. J Clin Endocrinol Metab. 2003;88:4525-4532.

136. Sandvik, L, Erikssen, J, Thaulow, R, Erikssen, G, Mundal, R, Rodahl, K. Physical fitness as a predictor of mortality among healthy, middle-aged Norwegian men. N Engl J Med. 1993;328:533-537.

137. Schnyder, G, Roffi, M. Flammer, Y, Pin, R, Hess, OM. Effect of homocysteine-lowering therapy with folic acid, vitamin B12, and vitamin B6 on clinical outcome after percutaneous coronary intervention: the Swiss Heart Study: a randomized controlled trial. JAMA. 2002;288:973-979.

138. Seman, LJ, DeLuca, C, Jenner, JL, Cupples, LA, McNamara, JR, Wilson, PWF, Castelli, WP, Ordovas, JM, Schaefer, EJ. Lipoprotein(a)-cholesterol and coronary heart disease in the Framingham Heart Study. Clin Chem. 199;45:1039-1046.

139. Sikand, G, Kashyap, ML, Yang, I. Medical nutrition therapy lowers serum cholesterol and saves medication costs in men and hypercholesterolemia. J Am Diet Assoc. 1998;98:889-894.

140. Simopoulos, Artemis, P., Merbert, Victor, and Jacobson, Beverly: *Genetic Nutrition*, MacMillan and Publishing Company, 866 Third Avenue, New York, N.Y. 10022, 1993.

141. Singer, P. Diagnosis of primary hyperlipoproteinemias. Z Gesamte Inn Med. 1977;32:129-133.

142. Singh, RB, Dubnov, G, Niaz, MA, Ghosh, S, Singh, R, Rastogi, SS, Manor, O, Pella, D, Berry, EM. Effect of an Indo-Mediterranean diet on progression of coronary artery disease in high-risk patients (Indo-Mediterranean Diet Heart Study): a randomized single-blind trial. Lancet. 2002;260:1455-1461.

143. Snoden, CB, McNamara, PM, Garrison, RJ, Feinleib, M, Kannel, WB, Epstein, FH. Predicting coronary heart disease in siblings – a multivariate assessment: the Framingham Heart Study. Am J Epidemiol. 1982;115:217-222.

144. Stehouwer, CDA, Weijenberg, MP, van den Berg, M, Jakobs, C, Feskens, EJM, Kromhout, D. Serum homocysteine and risk of coronary heart disease and cerebrovascular disease in elderly men: a 10-year follow-up. Arterioscler Thromb Vasc Biol. 1998;18:1895-1901.

145. Stern, MP, Haffner, SM. Body fat distribution and hyperinsulinemia as risk factors for diabetes and cardiovascular disease. Arteriosclerosis. 1986;6:123-130.

146. Stubbs, P, Seed, M, Lane, D, Collinson, P, Kendall, F, Noble, M. Lipoprotein(a) as a risk predictor for cardiac mortality in patients with acute coronary syndromes. Eur Heart J. 1998;19:1355-1364.

147. Steinbert, D. Low density lipoprotein oxidation and its pathobiological significance. J Biol Chem. 1997;272:20963-20966.

148. *The Surgeon General's Report on Nutrition and Health*, U.S. Department of Health and Human Services, DHHS (PHS) Publication No. 88-50210, 1988.

149. Thomas, I, Gupta, S, Sempros, C, Cooper, R. Serum lipids of Indian physicians living in the US compared to US-born physicians. Atherosclerosis. 1986;61:99-106.

150. Utermann, G. The mysteries of lipoprotein(a). Science. 1993;246:904-910.

151. Valkonen, M, Kuusi, T. Passive smoking induces atherogenic changes in low-density lipoprotein. Circulation. 1998;97:2012-2016.

152. Van Oort, FV, Melse-Boonstra, A, Brouwer, IA, Clarke, R, West, CE, Katan, MB, Verhoef, P. Folic acid and reduction in plasma homocysteine concentrations in older adults: a dose-response study. Am J Clin Nutr. 2003;77:1318-1323.

153. Van Horn, L, McDonald, A, Peters, E, Gernhofer, N. Dietary management of cardiovascular disease: a year 2002 perspective. Nutr Clin Care. 2001;4:314-331.

154. van den Hoogen, PCW, Feskens, EJM, Nagelkerke, NJD, Menotti, A, Nissinen, A, Kromhout, D, for the Seven Countries Research Group. The relation between blood pressure and mortality due to coronary heart disease among men in different parts of the world. N Engl J Med. 2000;342:1-8.

155. Vega, GL. Obesity, metabolic syndrome, and cardiovascular disease. Am Heart J. 2001;142:1108-1116.

156. Vikram, NK, Pandev, RM, Sharma, R, Misra, A. Hyperhomocysteinemia in healthy Asian Indians. Am J Hematol. 2003;72:151-152.

157. Vikram, NK, Misra, A, Dwivedi, M, Sharma, R, Pandey, RM, Luthra, K, Chatterjee, A, Dhingra, V, Jaikhani, BL, Talwar, KK, Guleria, R. Correlations of C-reactive protein levels with anthropometric profile, percentage of body fat and lipids in healthy adolescents and young adults in urban North India. Atherosclerosis. 2003;168:305-313.

158. Vermeulen, EG, Stehouwer, CD, Valk, J. Van Der Knaap, M. Van Den Berg, M, Twisk, JW, Prevoo, W, Rauwerda, JA. Effect of homocysteine-lowering treatment with folic acid plus vitamin B6 on progression of subclinical atherosclerosis: a randomized, placebo-controlled trial. Lancet. 2000;355:517-522.

159. Weverling-Rijnsburger, AW, Jonker, IJ, van Exel E, Gussekloo, J, Westendrop, RG. High-density vs low-density lipoprotein cholesterol as the risk factor for coronary artery disease and stroke in old age. Arch Intern Med. 2003;163:1549-1554.

160. Willett, WC, Green, A, Stampfer, MJ, Speizer, FE, Colditz, GA, Rosner, B, Monson, RR, Stason, W, Hennekens, CH. Relative and absolute excess risks of coronary heart disease among women who smoke cigarettes. N Engl J Med. 1987;317:1303-1309.

161. Wilson, PW, Garrison, RJ, Castelli, WP, Feinleib, M, McNamara, PM, Kannel, WB. Prevalence of coronary heart disease in the Framingham Offspring Study: role of lipoprotein cholesterols. Am J Cardiol. 1980;46:649-654.

162. Ximmet, P, Boyko, EJ, Collier, GR, de Courten, M. Etiology of the metabolic syndrome: potential role of insulin resistance, leptin resistance, and other players. Ann NY Acad Sci. 1999;892:25-44.

163. Yagalla, MV, Hoerr, SL, Song, WO, Enas, E, Garg, A. Relationship of diet, abdominal obesity, and physical activity to plasma lipoprotein levels in Asian Indian physicians residing in the United States. J Am Diet Asssoc. 1996;96:257-261.

ABBREVIATIONS

ADA	American Dietetic Association
AHA	American Heart Association
ALT	Alanine Aminotransferase
AST	Aspartate Aminotransferase
ATP III	Adult Treatment Panel of the National Cholesterol Education Program
BMI	Body Mass Index
CAD	Coronary Artery Disease
CHD	Coronary Heart Disease
CRP	C-Reactive Protein
CSFII	Continuing Survey of Food Intakes by Individuals
CVD	Cardiovascular Disease
DAG	Docosahexaenoic Acid
DASH	Dietary Approaches to Stop Hypertension
EPA	Eicosapentaenoic Acid
FDA	Food and Drug Administration
GI	Glycemic Index
GTP	Gamma-Glutamyltranspeptidase
HDL	High-Density Lipoprotein
IR	Insulin Resistance
JNC7	Joint National Committee on Prevention, Detection, Evaluation, and Treatment of High Blood Pressure
LDL	Low-Density Lipoprotein
LRC	Lipid Research Clinics Study
MES	Metabolic Syndrome
MI	Myocardial Infarction
MNT	Medical Nutrition Therapy
MRFIT	Multiple Risk Factor Intervention Trial
MSG	Monosodium Glutamate
MTHFR	Methyl Tetrahydrofolate Reductase
NASH	Nonalcoholic Steatohepatitis
NCEP	National Cholesterol Education Program Adult Treatment Panel III
NCEP	National Cholesterol Education Program
NCWR	National Weight Control Registry
NHLBI	National Heart, Lung, and Blood Institute
PPAR	Peroxisome Proliferator-Activated Receptor
PTCA	Percutaneous Transluminal Coronary Angioplast
TG	Triglyceride
TLC	Therapeutic Lifestyle Changes
VA-HIT	Veteran Affairs High-Density Lipoprotein Intervention Study
VLDL	Very-low-density Lipoprotein
VO2	Maximum Oxygen Uptake

Index

G

H

I

J

L

M

N

O

ABOUT THE AUTHOR
Lalita Kaul, PhD, RD, LD, LN

Dr. Kaul received her PhD from the University of Maryland. She is Professor of Nutrition in the Department of Community and Family Medicine, College of Medicine, Howard University (HU), Washington, DC. Dr. Kaul teaches medical students, residents and other health professionals.

Her area of expertise includes hypertension, overweight, obesity, cancer, diabetes, cardiovascular disease, hyperlipidemia, vegetarianism, and general nutrition. In addition, she has taught nutrition in several settings and has provided leadership for National and International conferences. She is the Director of Bariatric Clinic and has published over 40 papers. She is a member of Sigma XI, American Dietetic Association (ADA), NY Academy of Science, American Institute of Nutrition, American Institute of Clinical Nutrition, North American Association for the Study of Obesity and American Diabetes Association. She is listed in Who's Who in Diabetes Treatment, Education and Research. She is on the Editorial Board of the Journal of Nutrition for the Elderly. She has received several grants for nutritional studies. She has also conducted workshops on obesity for lay people.

Dr. Kaul is the National Spokesperson for The American Dietetic Association. She has been interviewed by news media about ADA's position on various diets and nutritional issues. Recently she was interviewed by the Washington Post about Chocolates and the importance of breakfast. She was also interviewed by the Washington Times about soft drinks in the schools. Recently she has published a book on obesity, *Multidisciplinary Approach to Obesity*. The book has been received very well.

In the past, she has worked in the White House Health Care Information Center and Presidential Correspondence Analysis. She was also a consultant at NIH. She was a pioneer in incorporating nutrition education in the medical curriculum at Howard University. She also developed a program for primary care physicians.

Printed in the United States
71333LV00002B/3-6

9 781596 637566